INTERVENTIONAL FLUOROSCOPY

INTERVENTIONAL FLUOROSCOPY

Physics, Technology, Safety

STEPHEN BALTER

Chapter Contributors

JACK T. CUSMA
Image Compression

JOHAN H. C. REIBER
Quantitative Coronary Angiography

MICHAEL D. O'HARA
Radiobiology

LOUIS K. WAGNER
Deterministic Radiation Effects

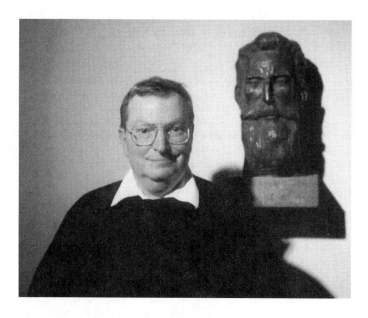

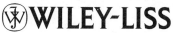**WILEY-LISS**

A John Wiley & Sons, Inc., Publication
New York • Chichester • Weinheim • Brisbane • Singapore • Toronto

Title page shows author at the Roentgen Museum, Wurtzburg, November 8, 1995. This photo was taken exactly 100 years later in the place that X-rays were discovered.

This book is printed on acid-free paper. ⊗

Library of Congress Cataloging-in-Publication Data:

Interventional fluoroscopy: physics, technology, and safety / Stephen Balter.
    p. cm.
   Includes bibliographical references and index.
   ISBN 0-471-39010-0 (cloth : alk. paper)
    1. Interventional radiology.   2. Interventional radiology—Safety measures.   3. Diagnosis, Fluoroscopic.   4. Diagnosis, Fluoroscopic—Safety measurs.   I. Balter, Stephen.
  RD33.55 .I575 2001
  617'.05—dc21
                                    00-043394

Printed in the United States of America.

10 9 8 7 6 5 4 3 2 1

To F. Mason Sones, Jr., M.D., founding father of coronary angiography.

He was my teacher, colleague, and friend.

With many cherished memories of times both on and off the job.

Much of the contents of this book originated in explaining radiation physics and fluoroscopic technology in response to his insatiable curiosity as to how his tools worked. What clarity is present in this writing was positively influenced by his continuous insistence on reducing the "fog-index" of manuscripts.

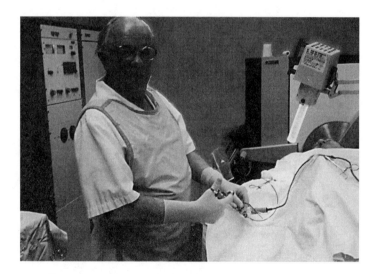

Contents

Foreword

We are living in an era in which an increasing number of diagnostic and therapeutic procedures are performed in the interventional laboratory. Whereas 20 years ago the specialist in catheterization was most likely a dedicated full-time angiographer, the dissemination of interventional techniques and the proliferation of laboratories has resulted in many "jacks of all trades" working in the interventional environment. This has lead to an interesting conundrum: interventional procedures are becoming increasingly complex and lengthy, whereas awareness by the average interventionalist of the specific techniques and issues of radiological vascular imaging is in decline. This has been compounded by the fact that current trainees derive much of their knowledge from a cohort of trainers, themselves not well acquainted with basic radiological principles.

There are several compelling reasons why this trend should be reversed. First, the issue of radiation safety in the angiographic suite is currently being reexamined by governmental regulatory bodies. Second, technological advances in the fields of image formation, storage, and retrieval are rapidly being incorporated into clinical practice. Interventionalists need a sound foundation in basic principles to grasp the meaning of these changes and to assess the relevance of these new technologies to their particular environment. Additionally, the emergence of vascular brachytherapy requires a new level of understanding of the risk/reward ration of therapeutic ionizing radiation. Only with an understanding of the principles of ionizing radiation, its biological effects, and attendant safety issues can the interventionalist begin to evaluate the place of this important therapeutic adjunct into the scheme of patient care. Finally, the emergence of subspecialty boards requiring specific curricula on radiological imaging and safety has helped raise the medical community's consciousness of these issues.

Dr. Balter is uniquely qualified to assemble this unique text. He has been involved in the field of radiological imaging and safety since the early days of coronary angiography, working with pioneers such as Melvin Judkins and Mason Sones. He also brings a practical perspective to this text in that he is a physicist who has spent a great deal of time with interventionalists and is acutely aware of the specific challenges that they confront in daily practice.

This book encompasses the breath of contemporary knowledge relevant to radiological imaging and safety and is organized into coherent and understandable chapters. In can be read in sequence or, more likely, be used as a constant reference for interventionalists to "bone up" on specific questions and problems that they confronted in the laboratory. Whether you are a laboratory directory, a full-time interventionalist, a clinical practitioner making occasional visits to the lab, or a fellow, the contents of this book represent an essential body of knowledge. Having it all in a single volume is an important step in promoting radiological literacy. I congratulate Dr. Balter and his colleagues on this effort.

J. W. Moses, M.D.
New York, New York

Introduction

The fluoroscope provides X-ray vision to the interventionalist. As fluoroscopically aided clinical tasks grow in complexity, imaging equipment manufacturers supply systems that are simultaneously highly automated (to minimize the operator's work load) and flexible (to maximize the application range of the equipment). The operator's understanding of imaging technology is essential to maximizing the utility of this tool while simultaneously reducing its risks. The focus of this book is therefore directed to the needs of the clinical interventionalist.

Section one reviews the basic physical and dosimetric concepts common to all X-ray projection imaging systems. Special attention is drawn to several words (e.g., contrast, dose), which are used in very different ways in technical and clinical arenas.

Section two presents an overview of the key components comprising interventional fluoroscope systems. Systems are highly integrated. This includes an extensive network of feedback and control circuits. The result is a flexible system capable of doing much more than was possible in the early 1990s.

Section three introduces the digital image and associated tools. Modern interventional fluoroscopes are essentially digital devices. Chapters on image compression and quantitative angiography are included.

Section four focuses on radiation safety issues. The use of ionizing radiation is extremely beneficial but not entirely benign. Constituencies who need to be considered include patients, laboratory staff, and the public. The section begins with chapters on basic radiation biology and radiation effects. It goes on to discuss operational means to manage radiation risk and the influences of the ever-present regulatory authority. The section ends with a brief introduction to an emerging interventional tool: Endovascular brachytherapy presents its own set of technological issues. This modality must be understood before it can be safely and effectively used.

The fifth and final section gives a brief overview of interventional fluoroscopic quality assurance. As in all areas of medicine, there is a need to independently verify the performance of clinical tools. This is complicated by the variability of interventional procedures and of clinical requirements. A newly approved phantom, developed by consensus between the interventional cardiology community and the medical imaging manufacturers, is presented as a tool meeting these needs.

The book itself provides breath of coverage. A selected bibliography provides pointers to additional depth of material.

Acknowledgments

Thanks are extended to the generation of students whose questions crystallized the topics and methods of presentation. Additional thanks are offered to colleagues in academia, industry, and clinical practice for their intellectual curiosity, critical comments, and encouragement.

This book originated as a series of tutorial articles that were inspired by Fred Heupler and commissioned by Frank Hildner. The draft chapters were reviewed and polished by numerous interactions with many colleagues at Lenox Hill.

Special thanks go to Cliff Double and Peter Marsden of the British Medical Device Agency for their critical review of the manuscript.

SECTION ONE

Physics

1

Radiation Concepts

ELECTROMAGNETIC RADIATION

X rays are a form of electromagnetic radiation. The main characteristics of X rays are similar to visible light. Radiation is conveniently discussed in terms of photons. A single photon is a quantum (discrete packet) of electromagnetic radiation containing a defined amount of energy. A stronger source produces more photons per second than a weaker source.

It takes thousands of X-ray photons per square millimeter to form a single fluoroscopic frame

A single X-ray quantum contains many thousands of times as much energy as does a visible light quantum. A green light photon contains two electron volts (eV) of energy. A typical germicidal ultraviolet (UV) photon has three electron volts of energy. A UV photon carries sufficient energy to produce ions by breaking molecular bonds. Those X-ray photons used for imaging have energies ranging from 10 keV (10,000 eV) up to 150 keV. The difference in biological effects between visible light and X rays is largely attributable to the difference in quantum energy content.

A "light" source such as a candle or X-ray tube converts input energy (chemical or electrical) into electromagnetic quanta. Another portion of the input energy heats the source. Radiation is the transport of energy away from the source by electromagnetic quanta. For the purpose of this chapter, we assume that the radiation is isotropic (uniformly emitted in all directions).

Picture a small candle in the center of a large space. Its flame can be considered a mathematical point. We artificially simplify our model if we assume that each light photon has the same energy. In Figure 1-1, all of the light energy emitted by the candle initially passes through the small inner sphere and then passes through the large outer sphere.

The light energy uniformly paints the surface of each sphere. Because the total amount of energy leaving the candle in one second is constant, the paint has to be spread thinner over the larger surface area of the outer sphere than

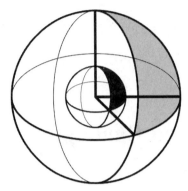

FIG. 1-1. Energy flow. All of the energy generated by a point source of radiation passes through each sphere in turn.

the smaller surface of the inner sphere. The intensity of the radiation (paint thickness) is the total energy (or number of quanta) produced by the candle in 1 s divided by the surface area of a particular sphere (Fig. 1-2). Radiation intensity is higher on spheres closer to the candle. Intensity can also be increased by using a brighter candle.

The energy content of a photon determines its color. When each of the photons in a light or X-ray beam has the same energy, the beam is called "monochromatic." A polychromatic beam contains photons with different energies. The energy carried by a beam is equal to the total energy of all of its photons. The spectrum of the beam is a histogram of the number of photons of each energy.

For convenience, a monochromatic beam is used in the remainder of this chapter. The beam energy is therefore equal to the total number of photons in the beam multiplied by the (single) energy carried by one photon. The intensity of the beam is measured by counting the number of photons crossing a small area in 1 s. At clinical imaging distances, the radii of the wedges in Figure 1-2 are so large that the surfaces are essentially planes. Consider a 1-

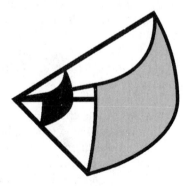

FIG. 1-2. Energy density. The energy density (intensity) is lower on the larger (outer) surface than it is on the smaller (inner) surface.

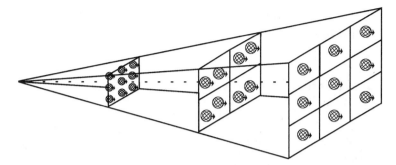

FIG. 1-3. Photon spread. The same number of photons passes through each of the three surfaces.

mm² patch located one meter from the source (Fig. 1-3). Let us assume that 900 photons pass through this patch in 1 s. At a distance of 2 m, the corresponding patch has a size of 4 mm². The 900 photons are now spread over a larger area. The photon density is now 900/4 = 225. The X-ray intensity is now reduced by a factor of four. This spreading of photons with increased distance from the source is expressed as the inverse square law. Continuing away from the source, at 3 m the area is now 9 mm² and the photon density is now 900/9 = 100. Tripling the distance reduces the intensity by a factor of nine.

A FIRST LOOK AT THE INTERACTION OF RADIATON AND MATTER

The physical interactions of an X-ray beam with a specific tissue are dependent both on the photon spectrum (the assortment of photon energies in the beam) and on the elemental composition and physical density of the tissue. Chemical bonding (energy levels of a few eV) has no appreciable influence on the absorption of diagnostic X rays (energy levels of several tens of keV). At an atomic level, the details depend on the energy of an individual photon and the atomic number of a single atom. These effects and their influence on image appearance are discussed in Chapter 3.

The distribution of interactions and energy deposition is very uneven at an atomic level. There are interactions with some atoms and no interactions with their neighbors. Radiation methodology works with what might be termed a "fat point." The measuring volume is simultaneously large enough to average out energy deposition fluctuations and small enough so that beam intensity is essentially uniform across the volume. Millimeter size volumes of tissue are large enough to meet this criterion for diagnostic X rays. This averaging is implicit in the following discussions of measurements "at a point."

RADIATON UNITS AND QUANTITIES

This section briefly introduces the radiation quantities found in the International System of units (SI units). These quantities, and their relationships, comprise the remainder of this chapter. The relationships between SI units themselves and between newer and older (almost obsolete) radiation units are given in the Appendix.

Dose (Concentration of Energy Delivered to Tissue)

The key quantity is "dose." It is a measure of the concentration of energy absorbed by tissue. The formal definition of dose is the amount of energy absorbed from the radiation field at a point divided by the mass of material at that point. The SI unit of dose is the gray (Gy).

1 gray (Gy) = 1 joule (of energy) absorbed per kilogram of a

specified material

Remembering that dose is a concentration, the averaging is over the "point" discussed in the previous section. The "point" needed to define dose in tissue for diagnostic X rays only contains a few milligrams of matter. A dose of 1 Gy means that each such point absorbs a few microjoules of energy.

A gray is a large unit. Radiation therapy doses are in the gray range. A surprisingly small amount of energy is deposited in tissue during medical procedures. For example, a dose of 2 Gy is usually delivered to a tumor in a single radiation therapy treatment. This means that 2 joules (J) of energy are delivered per kilogram of tissue. Assuming, for the moment, that water is equivalent to tissue, we would find the temperature rise to be 0.0005°C. It would take a few days to boil a cup of water at typical therapy dose rates. A lethal whole-body dose of radiation is less than 0.1 food calories of energy (about the heat content of a spoonful of coffee). Imaging doses are much lower. For example, a chest radiograph delivers a dose of approximately 100 μGy to the entrance skin.

Radiation dose is delivered by the interactions of photons with individual atoms. Direct biological response is localized to the point of interaction. The systemic effects seen during radiation treatments for cancer are secondary physiological responses stimulated by injured tissue.

Dose Equivalent (H)

In the big picture of radiation and its effects, different types and energies of radiation produce different biological effects for the same physical dose. The quantity "dose equivalent" accounts for this by means of an experimentally determined quality factor. The quality factor for diagnostic X-ray energies is one. The quality factor for other forms of radiation can range up to 20. The unit of dose equivalent is the sievert (Sv). Thus

1 sievert (Sv) = 1 Gy × Quality Factor

Exposure (Strength of the Radiation Field At A Given Point)

It is very difficult to directly measure the amount of radiation energy absorbed by a tissue sample. Most SI "exposure" measurements are actually measurements of air dose. This is reasonable because the absorption properties of a gram of air are similar to those of a gram of soft tissue.

"Exposure" is the measure of an X-ray beam's ability to ionize air. The absorbed energy causes this. The SI unit of exposure is the coulomb (unit of electrical charge) per kilogram of air. This unit has not been generally accepted for routine work.

The current working unit of exposure is air-kerma. Air-kerma is a measure of the energy extracted from the beam by air This mouthful translates as the Kinetic Energy Released per Unit MAss of air. The unit of measurement is the gray (Gy) (1 joule per kilogram of *air*). In obsolescent units, exposure is measured in Roentgens (R). This is a measure of the ionization produced per gram of air. An air-kerma of 1 Gy corresponds to an exposure of 114 R.

Some instruments directly measure the ionization produced in a defined volume of air. These instruments are called ionization chambers (Fig. 1-4). Because the elemental composition of air is close to soft tissue, these instruments provide an accurate representation of soft tissue dose. Other types of instruments, such as Geiger counters (Fig. 1-5), can detect the presence of radiation but are not particularly suitable for dose measurements.

Ionization chamber probes come in different sizes. Larger chambers collect the larger total amount of ionization produced in the larger measuring volume. A larger chamber produces a stronger signal in exchange for reduced spatial resolution. Part of the art of radiation dosimetry is matching the ionization chamber to the immediate measurement task.

It is useful to describe the distribution of radiation intensity at various places in the laboratory. This is done by measuring the amount of air ionization produced by radiation at those locations. These are called "exposure" measurements. ("Exposure" is a word with a specific dosimetric meaning that differs somewhat from common usage.)

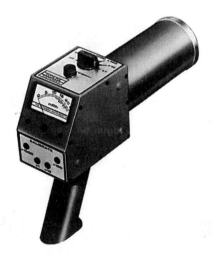

FIG. 1-4. Ionization chamber survey meter. This instrument is used to measure exposure rates. The ion chamber is the cylindrical structure to the right. [Photograph courtesy of Nuclear Associates.]

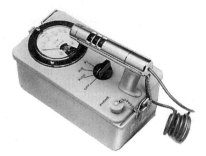

FIG. 1-5. Geiger counter. This instrument is used as a radiation detector. The GM detector element is shown attached to the handle. [Photograph courtesy of Nuclear Associates.]

Exposure in a formal dosimetric context has nothing to do with anybody being affected by radiation. Exposure is not dose (Fig. 1-6). Exposure describes the amount of radiation at a point in space. This radiation field can deliver dose to tissue or other materials. The amount of dose delivered to a small volume of tissue depends on both the strength of the radiation field and the nature of the interaction of the radiation field with the local tissue.

Dose Distributions

Figure 1-7 schematically illustrates the extraction of energy from a beam and its deposition at a point. Radiation enters the small mass. Some of this energy is locally absorbed, and the remainder leaves the mass via a variety of physical processes. In the illustration, 8 J enters the mass. Three joules are absorbed by

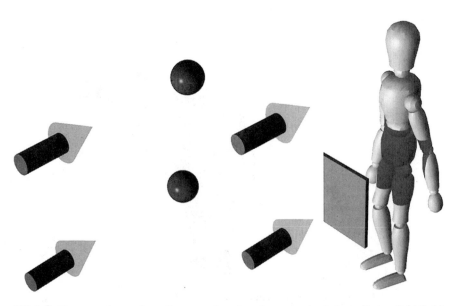

FIG. 1-6. Exposure is not dose. Exposure describes the strength of the radiation field (left). Dose describes the amount of energy received by a small volume of tissue.

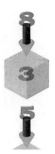

FIG. 1-7. Dose. Net energy absorbed at a "point."

the material in the cube. The remaining energy (5 J) leaves the cube. We further simplify this drawing by assuming that all of the emerging energy leaves the cube at its bottom. Note that the numbers used in this discussion are exaggerated for teaching purposes. In reality, a dosimetric equilibrium point will extract a very small fraction of 1% of the incoming beam's energy. A portion of the extracted energy is absorbed by the material in the cube. Physical scattering processes also direct another small fraction of the incoming energy into multiple directions.

Figure 1-8 illustrates a larger volume of tissue irradiated by a uniform X-ray beam. The same amount of energy enters each of the small cubes on the entrance surface (8 J per cube). The total X-ray energy entering the entire mass of tissue increases as the beam size increases. In this illustration, the beam irradiates nine cubes when it first enters the tissue. The total energy entering the tissue is therefore $8 \times 9 = 72$.

Some of the radiation energy in the beam is absorbed in each layer of the tissue. In Figure 1-8, 2 J emerge from each of the nine cubes in the bottom layer. The total radiation energy leaving the tissue is therefore $2 \times 9 = 18$. The total energy absorbed by the tissue is the difference between the energy in and the energy out (54 J). Direct biological effects of radiation on tissue are *not* simply related to the total energy delivered. The actual effect is determined by the type of tissue in each cube and the actual amount of energy absorbed by that small bit of tissue.

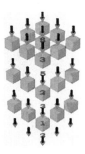

FIG. 1-8. Energy fluence. The total amount of energy entering this volume of matter is equal to the energy entering each of the top cubes multiplied by the number of cubes in the top row.

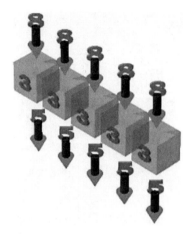

FIG. 1-9. Row of "dose" cubes. One row of the elementary cubes on the entrance surface of the volume shown in Fig. 1-8.

Figure 1-9 illustrates one row of identical cubes on the entrance surface of the tissue. The same dose is delivered to each cube because the mass and amount of energy absorbed in each cube is identical.

Figure 1-10 illustrates one column of identical cubes extending through the thickness of the tissue. Each cube in the column absorbs some of the entering energy and transmits the remainder. Energy absorbed in an upper cube is not available to irradiate lower cubes. The dose delivered to the top cube is higher than that delivered to the middle cube. Even less dose is delivered to the bottom cube. For imaging X rays, half of the total beam energy is absorbed in the first few centimeters of tissue. This is why superficial tissues on the entrance surface of the patient are at greatest risk.

Often times, one finds the term "organ dose" in the literature (e.g., the thyroid dose from a procedure was 23 Gy). This is a shorthand way of saying

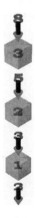

FIG. 1-10. Column of "dose" cubes. One column of elementary cubes through the volume shown in Fig 1-8. Less energy enters each successive cube because of absorption by the upper cubes.

that the actual dose delivered to each bit of tissue in that organ is more or less the same and is equal to the stated value. It is extremely difficult to deliver the same dose to all of the tissues in a human being. Therefore, the phrase "radiation dose delivered to a patient" is usually an incorrect usage. Also, a film-badge reading (measured at the collar) does not really represent a uniform dose delivered to all of the tissues of its wearer.

DOSE AREA PRODUCT MEASUREMENT

Modern cardiac fluoroscopes may include a built-in "dosimeter." Many of these instruments actually measure air-kerma area product. For historical reasons, these instruments are called dose area product (DAP) meters. Dose and DAP are *not* interchangeable. Dose refers to the energy locally absorbed by a small mass of tissue. It is used to predict the biological response of that bit of tissue. DAP essentially refers to the total X-ray energy leaving the X-ray tube. It is used to estimate the cancer risk to the patient and the amount of scatter in the lab.

Figure 1-11 illustrates a single layer of absorber divided into 1-cm cubes. Each cube face has a surface area of 1 cm^2. Imagine, for the moment, that all the X-ray energy in the beam is absorbed in this one layer (we will discuss the effects in tissue below). Each of the 25 cubes shown in Figure 1-11 receives the same dose (3 Gy). In this case, the DAP is equal to 3 Gy $\times$ 25 cm^2 = 75 Gycm^2.

In Figure 1-12 the beam has been collimated so that only nine cubes are irradiated. The corresponding DAP is now 3 Gy $\times$ 9 cm^2 = 27 Gycm^2. In Figure 1-13, the beam intensity has been doubled. The DAP is now 6 $\times$ 9 = 54 Gycm^2.

In the interventional laboratory, essentially all of the X-ray energy in the useful beam is absorbed somewhere in the patient. A superficial layer of tissue will only absorb a fraction of the beam energy. However, the total tissue thickness in the beam path is sufficient to absorb the rest. A first approximation to cancer induction is to assume that the risk is proportional to total energy absorption. (A better approximation includes knowledge of the distribution of

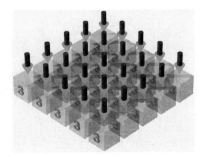

FIG. 1-11. Example of dose area product (DAP). The dose delivered to each 1 cc cube is 3 Gy. The DAP is 75 Gycm^2. Each cube absorbs less energy than the injury threshold.

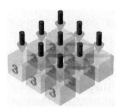

FIG. 1-12. Collimated beam. The beam is collimated to 9 cubes. The DAP is now 27 Gycm^2. Each cube receives the same dose as the corresponding cube in Fig 1-11.

dose within the patient and the radiosensitivity of individual tissues.) Estimating radiogenic cancer risk is a major reason why the public health authorities in some countries mandate total DAP measurements. "DAP" usually refers to the total energy passing through the measuring instrument.

In Figure 1-11, each tissue cube on the patient's surface receives 3 Gy from the beam. This is below the threshold for major skin injury (refer to Chapter 12 for skin dose injury levels). If the beam area is increased from 9 to 25 cm^2 (compare Figs. 1-11 and 1-12), then more skin is irradiated. The dose delivered to each bit of irradiated skin remains the same. However, if the intensity of the beam is doubled (Fig. 1-13), the dose delivered to each bit of irradiated skin is also doubled. In this example, the skin injury threshold has been exceeded. This happens even though more total energy was applied to the patient through the large field.

DAP is easier to measure than "skin dose." The radiation detector in a DAP meter is a very large ionization chamber. This is usually placed in the X-ray tube housing. The chamber size is large enough to totally intercept the X-ray beam.

Picture, if you will, that the ionization chamber volume is divided into a layer of cubes similar to those shown in Figure 1-11. The beam size determines the total number of irradiated cubes. The beam intensity determines the energy delivered to each cube. The total energy delivered to the ionization chamber by the beam is therefore the product of the number of irradiated cubes and the energy delivered to the air contained in any one cube.

The transmission ionization chamber used for DAP measurements (Fig. 1-14) is constructed in a way that minimizes its own absorption of radiation.

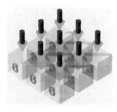

FIG. 1-13. High intensity. The entrance beam intensity has been doubled. The DAP is now 54 Gycm^2. However, 6 Gy is absorbed in each cube. (This is above the injury threshold.) Note that, even though the total DAP is less than the situation in Figure 1-11, the dose delivered to each of the nine cubes shown here is higher.

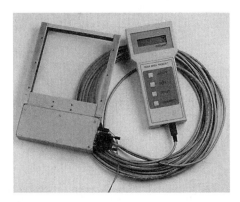

FIG. 1-14. DAP meter. The ion chamber is shown on the left and the readout electronics on the right.

Thus, almost all of the X-ray energy leaving the X-ray tube passes through the DAP chamber and is available to irradiate the patient.

As long as the DAP chamber is large enough to intercept the entire X-ray beam, its distance from the focal-spot is unimportant. As the chamber (refer back to Figs. 1-1 and 1-3) is moved away from the source of radiation, two effects occur: 1) The field size increases in proportion to the square of the distance from the source to the measuring location, and 2) the beam intensity decreases inversely with the square of the same distance. These two effects exactly offset each other (no surprise because the same total number of photons is available at either the near or far measuring position). Therefore, DAP is independent of measuring distance. Indeed, the DAP near the patient is the same as the DAP measured near the X-ray tube.

MINI COURSE

X rays are a form of electromagnetic radiation.

The intensity of an X-ray beam decreases inversely as the square of the distance between the source and measuring point.

Radiation dose is the amount of energy absorbed by a small mass of tissue (concentration).

2

Imaging Factors and Optimization

Angiographic imaging is optimized to maximize the visibility of anatomical structures containing contrast media.

Radiography is a form of projection imaging. The patient is illuminated with a source of X rays. The X-ray beam intensity is modulated by structures in the patient. This modulated beam is then detected by an image receptor. Characteristics of the image of a structure that affect its visibility are sharpness, contrast, and noise. Patient dose considerations affect the ability to optimize imaging parameters.

IMAGING GEOMETRY

Optical analogies illustrate many aspects of X-ray imaging. Let us start with the shadow of a thin coin cast by a point source of light on to a piece of paper (Fig. 2-1). A shadow is formed when some of the light rays are intercepted by the opaque coin. The shadow on the paper is larger than the coin. The shape of the shadow will be distorted if the coin is not parallel to the paper.

The focal spot of the X-ray tube replaces the point source of light. An image-receptor (e.g., film, image intensifier) replaces the paper. An artery or other structure replaces the coin. None of these items has the geometric precision of the optical experiment described in the previous paragraph. The selection of an imaging technique balances the effects of the physical nature of one of these items against those of another.

The nomenclature commonly used to describe radiographic imaging geometry is shown in Figure 2-2. The distance from the focal spot to the image receptor is called the source-to-image-receptor distance (SID). The distance from the object of interest to the image receptor is called the object-to-image-receptor distance (OID). The magnification of the object increases as the SID decreases or the OID increases.

15

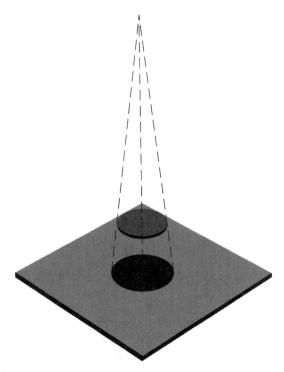

FIG. 2-1. Shadow imaging. The shadow of a coin cast by a point source of light is sharp (there is an abrupt change from light to dark) and magnified (the shadow is larger than the coin).

The distance from the focal spot to the patient's skin is called the source-to-skin distance (SSD). In general, increasing SSD decreases the patient's skin dose.

The distance between the exit surface of the patient and the image receptor is called the "gap" in this book. An excessive gap is often poor practice. Minimizing the gap is important in terms of both dose and image quality.

Angiographic fluoro systems usually have an isocentric mounting (Fig. 2-3). There may be one or two rotational axis. In a two-axis system, the beam rotates and skews around the patient in such a way that the central ray always passes through one fixed isocentric point. An object at isocenter remains in view as the beam moves. Operators usually place the artery or organ of interest at the isocenter to take advantage of this fact. In many systems, the source-to-isocenter distance (SAD) is fixed and the SID is adjustable. The magnification of an object at the isocenter increases as SID increases.

SHARPNESS

The shadow of the coin cast by a point source of light shown in Figure 2-1 is very sharp. There is an abrupt transition from the bright surroundings into the dark shadow. Two separate sharp shadows are cast by two separate point sources

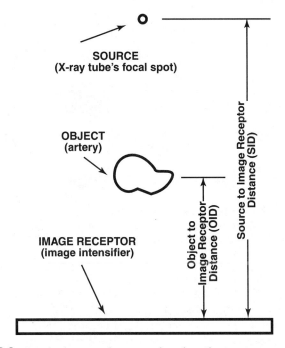

FIG. 2-2. Standard nomenclature used to describe imaging geometry.

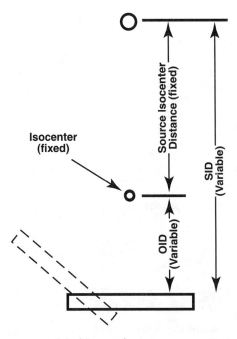

FIG. 2-3. Isocentric geometry. An object at the isocenter remains in view as the imaging system is rotated.

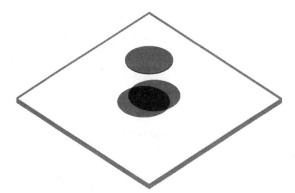

FIG. 2-4. **Overlapping shadows cast by two point sources of light.** Unshadowed areas on the screen are bright. Areas shadowed from both sources are dark. Areas shadowed from one source and illuminated by the other are gray.

(Fig. 2-4). The resulting shadow structure is complex. There is a region on the screen that remains dark because it is in the shadow of both sources. The surrounding region remains bright because it is in neither shadow. Two partially shadowed regions now appear. These are of intermediate brightness because they are illuminated by one source and shadowed by the other.

Penumbra

An extended light source can be thought of as a number of point sources (Fig. 2-5). The dark region remains (umbra). This area is in the shadow of all points in the extended source. The bright, unshadowed surrounding region remains. The annular transition region (penumbra) increases in brightness as one goes from the umbra to the surrounding. A wide penumbra produces an unsharp image. Penumbra increases as the size of the light source increases. As shown in Figure 2-6, penumbra also increases with magnification.

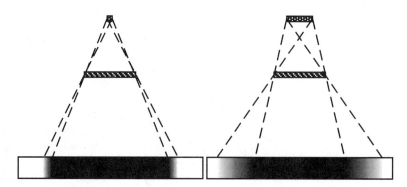

FIG. 2-5. **Overlapping shadows cast by an extended light source.** The fully shadowed area is the umbra. The partially shadowed region is the penumbra. Penumbra increases as source size increases.

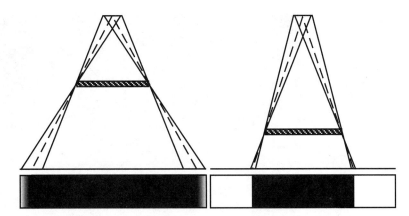

FIG. 2-6. Penumbra increases as magnification increases. At a magnification of ×2, the width of the penumbra is equal to the focal-spot size.

The focal spot of the X-ray tube is an extended light source. X rays are produced by bombarding the target with high-energy electrons. Extending the focal spot area eliminates overheating of the target and its literal melt down. Penumbra, caused by the size of the focal spot, is the first source of unsharpness in the image.

Motion Unsharpness

Objects can move while their picture is being taken. In Figure 2-7, a point source casts a shadow of a moving coin. The dark region is in shadow during the entire imaging time, and the bright surrounding is never shadowed. The transition region consists of those regions that are shadowed during a part of the imaging time. Faster moving objects produce more motion unsharpness.

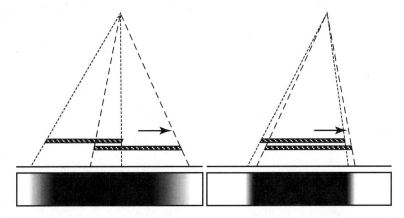

FIG. 2-7. Motion unsharpness. The moving coin shadows portions of the image receptor for part of the exposure time. The resulting brightness gradient gives unsharp images perpendicular to the direction of travel. Motion unsharpness increases as object velocity increases.

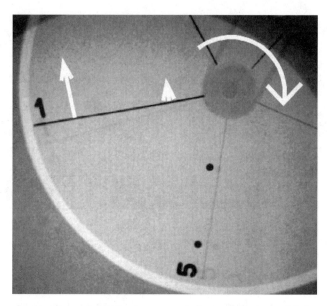

FIG. 2-8. **Image of moving wires.** The wires rotate about an axis near the upper right-hand corner. Parts of the wire closer to the axis have a smaller linear velocity than parts further from the axis The greater motion unsharpness produces increased blur. This is more easily seen on the fine wire (5). The "ghosts" are due to video lag. This effect is discussed in Chapter 6.

Figure 2-8 is the image of a rotating angiographic guide wire. The linear velocity of the wire increases at greater distances from the center of rotation. Portions of the wire toward the periphery of the disk have more motion blur than those portions nearer the center.

Reducing imaging time reduces motion unsharpness. However, rapid exposures require more X-ray tube power and therefore a larger focal spot. Sharpness is optimized by operating at the balance point that is relevant to the clinical task.

Receptor Blur

The image receptor further contributes to image unsharpness. Thick X-ray detectors are more dose efficient than thin detectors. There is also more radiation and light diffusion in a thick detector (Fig. 2-9).

CONTRAST

The word "contrast" has many meanings in radiological imaging. The appropriate meaning can usually be inferred from the context of the discussion.

An object can be detected when it contrasts with its surroundings. Two major factors contribute to the overall contrast of an object relative to its surroundings. These are "subject contrast" and "display contrast." These factors are

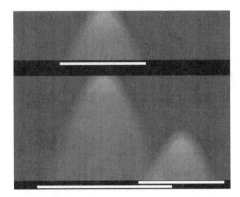

FIG. 2-9. Receptor blur. Thicker detectors are more efficient than thinner detectors. However, thick detectors often diffuse image edges more than thin detectors. Receptor blur is the third source of geometric unsharpness. The white bars illustrate the size of the blur pattern.

discussed in general terms in this chapter. The underlying physics and technology are discussed later in this book. When the patient is irradiated, different structures absorb different fractions of the beam. This produces the modulated X-ray beam that leaves the patient (Fig. 2-10). For example, iodine containing "contrast media" is used to enhance the visibility of vessels. Iodine works because it absorbs more of the radiation beam than the displaced blood. Carbon dioxide (CO_2) can also be used as a contrast medium. CO_2 works because

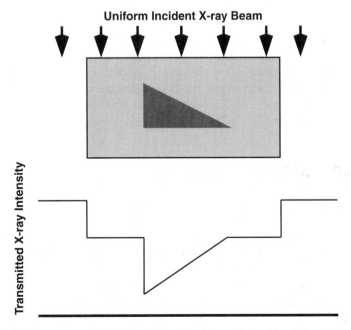

FIG. 2-10. Subject contrast. A uniform X-ray beam is modulated by differential absorption of radiation by different tissues.

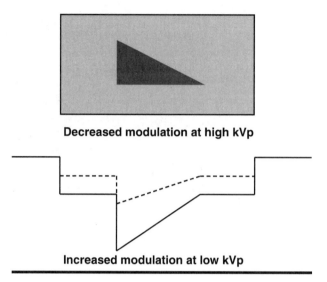

Decreased modulation at high kVp

Increased modulation at low kVp

FIG. 2-11. kVp affects contrast. High kVp beams produce less beam modulation than low kVp beams.

it absorbs less radiation than blood. The physics of subject contrast is discussed in Chapter 3.

Increasing the peak kilovolts (kVp) of an X-ray beam increases its penetrating power. For a given tissue thickness, patient dose decreases as kVp increases. The increased penetration is also used to examine thick body parts. However, increased kVp decreases the relative absorption of different tissues (Fig. 2-11). The net result is a decrease in beam modulation and subject contrast.

Tube voltage (kVp) can be maintained at an appropriate level by adjusting total tube power, exposure time, or detector sensitivity. Too much attention to subject contrast can result in decreased sharpness. Here, one sees the need to balance the requirement for contrast (needed to detect the object) and the requirement for sharpness (needed to characterize it).

SCATTERED RADIATION AND GRIDS

Scattered radiation is produced when the X-ray beam interacts with the patient (further information on X-ray interactions may be found in Chapter 3). Image contrast is reduced when scattered radiation reaches the image receptor. The amount of scatter increases with increases in the size of the X-ray field and the intensity of the X-ray beam (Fig. 2-12).

A radiographic grid reduces the amount of scatter reaching the image receptor. This type of grid is often called a "Bucky" grid after its inventor. As shown in Figure 2-13, the grid is placed between the patient and the image receptor. A grid consists of a series of lead strips and radiolucent interspaces. The lead strips are aimed to converge at the X-ray focal spot. Most of the

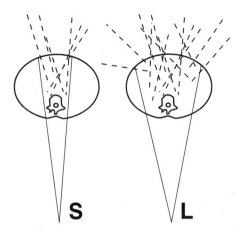

FIG. 2-12. Scatter production. Increases with field size and beam intensity. S = Small field, L = Large field size. (Only the scatter directed toward the image receptor is shown.)

image forming primary photons (see Fig. 2-13A) pass through the space between the lead strips.

A small fraction of the primary photons (Fig. 2-13B) are absorbed by the lead strips. Scattered radiation, produced in the patient, is less well directed than the primary beam. Most of these photons (C) have paths that pass through the lead strips. They are absorbed by the grid. Some scattered photons (D) pass through the interspaces and degrade image contrast. Other scattered photons (E) are directed out of the patient in other directions. The effects of scatter on the environment surrounding the interventional system are discussed in Chapter 13.

The efficiency of a grid is characterized by its grid ratio (Fig. 2-14) and its total lead content. A high ratio grid (e.g., 16:1) has a limited acceptance angle for scattered radiation. It also must be carefully positioned relative to

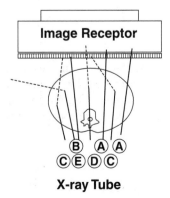

X-ray Tube

FIG. 2-13. Grid function. A: Primary photons passing through grid. B: Primary photon absorbed by grid strip. C: Scatter photons absorbed by grid strip. D: Scatter photon passing through grid. E: Scatter photon that misses image receptor.

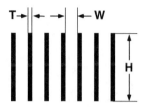

FIG. 2-14. Grid ratio (see text). Ratio = H/W (H = height of lead strips, W = width of interspace between lead strips, T = thickness of strips).

the focal spot of the X-ray tube. High ratio grids are suitable for high-kV radiography. Lower ratio grids (e.g., 8:1) are somewhat less efficient in scatter cleanup than higher ratio grids. They are more tolerant of changes in SID. Thus, low-ratio grids are found in interventional systems.

All grids absorb a fraction of the useful X-ray beam. In an ideal case, the primary beam transmission is given by

$$P = W/(T + W)$$

where W is the width of interspace between lead strips and T is the thickness of strips.

Real grids use aluminum, fiber, or plastic as an interspace material. The grids are also covered for mechanical protection. Any material absorbs some of the beam. This causes a small further reduction of primary beam transmission.

Grids are of little value for thin patients or body parts. Little scatter is produced in these circumstances. Here, removing the grid has little effect on image contrast. It does eliminate the primary beam losses. This results in a reduction of patient entrance dose.

Grid removal should also be considered while using magnification techniques. Moving the image receptor away from the patient reduces scatter degradation of the image. This is often called "air gap." Scatter reduction is due to a decrease of the solid-angle subtended by the image receptor not by air attenuation.

Display Contrast

The contrast in an electronic image can also be manipulated by adjusting the contrast controls on the display device. This is easy to do when working with a digital or video system (Fig. 2-15). Film users control display contrast by selecting a film type with appropriate characteristics.

NOISE

Reducing noise by increasing detector "dose" may increase the patient's effective dose and hence radiation risk.

There are point-to-point variations in the brightness of the radiographic image of a uniform plastic block. These fluctuations are called image noise. The main

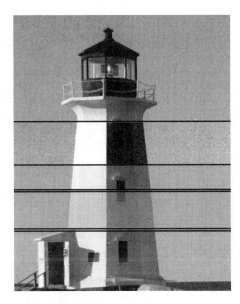

FIG. 2-15. Display contrast. Contrast can also be controlled by adjusting the display. Contrast is increased in the upper box (defined by the two single lines) and decreased in the lower box (defined by the two double lines).

sources of noise are the mechanical microstructure of the detector, electronic gain fluctuations, and the quantum nature of the X-ray beam. The first two factors have been reduced in importance by improved technology. However, because of fundamental physical factors, X-ray noise increases as the detector dose decreases.

Noise is the random fluctuation of image brightness. Contrast is the difference in image brightness between the shadow of an object and its surroundings. Noise reduces the ability to see low-contrast structures. Figures 2-16 and 2-17 present two images of the same patient taken using the same imaging system within 2 s. The difference in appearance is due to a 200:1 difference in the dose delivered to the image receptor.

THE BALANCE OF IMAGING FACTORS

Decreasing detector thickness to gain sharpness may make require more X-ray power to reduce noise to a tolerable level. The resulting sharpness gain may be negated by the need for a larger focal spot or a longer exposure time. The optimization balance (Fig. 2-18) has three arms: penumbra, exposure time, and receptor blur.

A simulation of the effect of detector thickness on sharpness is shown in Figure 2-19. The "original" image is shown in Fig. 2-19a. High- and low-contrast linear structures simulate vessels. High- and low-contrast simulated spheres represent objects such as chest nodules. All of these structures are shown as both black and white objects against a midtone background.

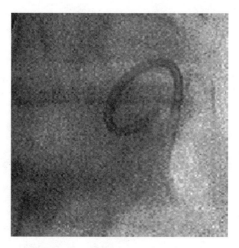

FIG. 2-16. **Low-dose clinical image.** This single-frame fluoroscopic last-image hold was acquired using a low detector dose.

Figure 2-19b simulates a thin detector and a finite quantity of radiation to image the object seen in Figure 2-19a. The continuity of the "vessels" allows both the high- and low-contrast targets to be seen in the presence of this degree of noise. The low-contrast "spheres" are lost in the noise.

Figure 2-19c simulates a thick detector and the same quantity of radiation used to form image Figure 2-19b. The "thick detector" blurs the noise. While doing this, it also blurs the "vessels" beyond recognition. However, the same blurring pulls the "spheres" back together and improves their visibility.

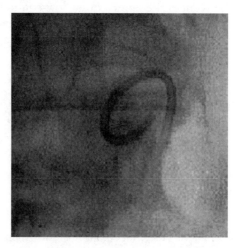

FIG. 2-17. **High-dose clinical image.** This digital fluorographic image was acquired a few seconds after the image shown Figure 2.13. The detector dose was approximately 200 times as high.

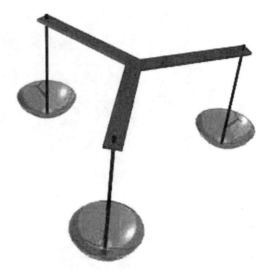

FIG. 2-18. Image quality balance. The sharpness balance has three arms: penumbra, motion, and receptor. All three are equal in an optimized imaging system. The balance can also be labeled with the arms being "sharpness," "contrast," and noise. Here the balance depends on the clinical task at hand.

This simulation represents the trade-off that was possible with film-screen systems. The "sharp" scenario in Figure 2-19b simulates thin intensifying screens used with a fast X-ray film. The "blurred" scenario in Figure 2-19c represents the use of thick intensifying screens and a slower X-ray film. In both cases, the dose delivered to the cassette is identical. The choice of films and screens was an important consideration in the film-changer era. One selected the combination appropriate for the majority of the patients expected in the laboratory. In the digital era, one can theoretically select the degree of sharpening or blurring appropriate to the task. However, some general balance is needed to minimize reading time.

The balance shown in Figure 2-18 can be relabeled to indicate that any given examination involves a balance between "sharpness," "contrast," and "noise." As can be seen from the simulations in Figure 2-19, there is no universal solution. The balance points depend on the clinical task. Interventional procedures usually need to maximize the visibility of relatively high-contrast objects. This can be done at the cost of increased visual noise and decreased low-contrast sensitivity.

MORE OPTIMIZATION

The visibility of noise can be reduced by spatial or temporal filtering. Spatial filtering reduces noise by averaging out the brightness variations around each point in the image. This is the equivalent of using an unsharp detector. Temporal filtering reduces noise by averaging the brightness variations at each

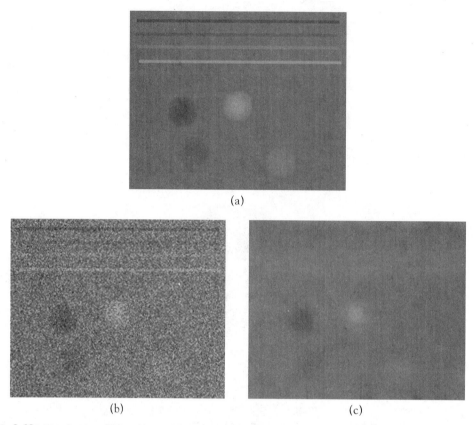

(a)

(b)   (c)

FIG. 2-19. Simulation of the effect of detector thickness (at constant detector "dose"). a (top): Simulation of the physical object. The linear structures represent vessels. The spherical objects represent nodules. Both sets of structures are present with high and low radiographic contrast. b (middle): Simulation of a thin detector and a finite image receptor dose. The low-contrast linear structures are easier to see against the noise than the low-contrast spheres. c (bottom); Simulation of a thick detector. The "dose" is identical to that in b. Receptor blur hides most of the noise and enhances the visibility of the spheres. The same process blurs the "vessels" to invisibility.

point in a series of images. This is the equivalent of using a long exposure time and can lead to motion unsharpness.

Image processing can be used to increase sharpness. Sharpening algorithms determine object edges by brightness variations. These algorithms also unavoidably increase the visibility of noise. Detector dose can be increased by increasing patient dose. This has consequences beyond the obvious one of increased patient risk. More X-ray energy is needed. Larger focal spots may be needed to handle the increased power. This increases penumbra. Longer exposure times increase motion unsharpness. Higher kVp increases penetration but decreases contrast.

Optimization of dose and image quality is task dependent. The three main image-quality parameters, sharpness, contrast, and noise, are interdependent in radiographic systems. The need to minimize patient dose imposes further couplings between these factors. This is the reason why there are no universally applicable imaging-systems.

MINI COURSE

An image represents a balance between sharpness, contrast, and noise.

Increasing subject contrast or reducing image noise usually increases patient and staff radiation risk.

The optimum balance of these factors is task specific. Interventional images are usually optimized to enhance the visibility of devices and contrast media.

3

X-Ray Physics

PHYSICS OF IMAGE FORMATION

An image is formed by differential attenuation of the X-ray beam. The physical mechanisms contributing to differential attenuation are differences in thickness (t), physical density [$\rho(g/cm^3)$], or atomic composition (Z). An initially uniform beam is modulated by structures possessing one or more or these differences (Fig. 3-1). Details of the attenuation coefficients of materials are discussed below. These coefficients have functional dependencies on the energy of the photon and the atomic number of the material.

The radiographic image of the chest is formed by all of these mechanisms. The portion of the beam passing through the liver experiences a greater thickness of tissue than the portion passing through the soft tissue of the shoulder. The lower physical density of a normal (air-containing) lung absorbs less radiation than the adjacent soft tissues of the mediastianum. The higher average atomic number of the calcium-containing ribs causes them to attenuate the beam to a degree disproportionate to their thickness and density.

The physical properties of an anatomic structure, such as an artery, are temporarily altered by injecting substances called "contrast media." Iodine is the active ingredient in most vascular agents. Iodine functions by altering the atomic composition of the filling of the artery. Carbon dioxide (CO_2) is also used as a contrast medium. CO_2 functions by altering the physical density of the vessel lumen. Optimum visualization of these two fundamentally different kinds of contrast media is achieved by selecting different settings of the X-ray imaging system.

SUBJECT CONTRAST

Subject contrast may be defined by comparing the intensity of an X-ray beam transmitted through a target relative to the transmission through its uniform surroundings (Fig. 3-2). In mathematical terms

31

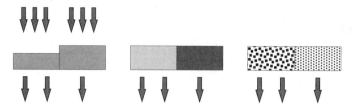

FIG. 3-1. Modulation of the X-ray beam. An X-ray beam can be modulated by differences in thickness, physical density, or atomic composition.

$$C_{subject} = I_t/I_b$$

Subject contrast is reduced by scattered radiation. The minimum usable net subject contrast for nonsubtracted images is around 2%. The primary limitation on minimum contrast is image noise.

$$C_{subject}^{with\ scatter} = (I_t + I_{scatter})/(I_b + I_{scatter})$$

$$C_{subject}^{with\ scatter} < C_{subject}$$

Radiographic grids (discussed in Chapter 2) are used to minimize the amount of scatter reaching the image receptor. There is a cost to the resulting improvement in subject contrast. The grid also absorbs some of the useful beam. This requires an increased irradiation of the patient and actually increases total scatter production.

Scatter production increases as the volume of irradiated tissue increases. Scatter is not a good thing. In addition to the loss of image quality, the stray radiation around an angiographic table is almost exclusively scatter.

Collimating the X-ray beam to the region of interest is a rare example of a win-win situation. The resulting reduction of scatter production improves the image and reduces staff exposure.

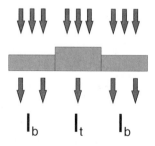

FIG. 3-2. Definition of subject contrast. In this drawing, subject contrast is created by a difference in thickness between the target and its surroundings.

X-RAY PRODUCTION

The technology of X-ray production is discussed in Chapter 4. This section introduces the relationship between the electrical factors applied to the X-ray tube and the resulting radiation output. These factors are the voltage applied across the X-ray tube [expressed as peak kilovolts (kVp)], the current flowing through the tube [expressed as milliamperes (mA)], and the time in which the current flows [expressed as seconds or milliseconds (s, ms)].

In this chapter, histograms are used to display the detailed properties of the X-ray beam. These histograms indicate the photon energy (in KeV) on the abscissa and the number of photons carrying an energy on the ordinate.

The rate of X-ray emission is proportional to the current flowing through the tube. The total quantity of emitted radiation is proportional to the current-time product. More radiation is emitted when the product of current and time (mAs) is increased (Fig. 3-3). This increases the numbers of photons at each energy in the spectrum. More radiation passing through the target produces a brighter image. However, the subject contrast between two objects remains the same.

Increasing kVp is more complex (Fig. 3-4). More photons are produced at each of the energies originally accessible. Photons are also produced at energies between the original and new kVp. The net effect on a fluoroscopic image is an increase in brightness and a decrease in subject contrast.

Increasing mA linearly increases X-ray production and leaves subject contrast unchanged.

Increasing kV superlinearly increases X-ray production and reduces subject contrast.

Figure 3-5 illustrates the spectrum of emitted X rays as a function of tube voltage. There is no emission at low energies because of self-filtration by elements of the tube. Additional filtration (discussed later in this chapter) is often

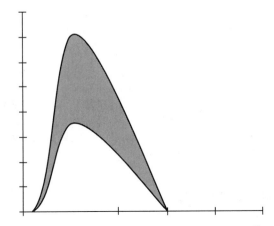

FIG. 3-3. Effect of tube current. Increasing tube current proportionally increases the number of photons produced at each energy.

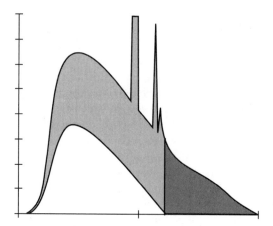

FIG. 3-4. Effect of tube voltage. Increasing tube voltage increases the number of photons produced at each energy in the original spectrum and produces additional photons at higher energies. Note the production of characteristic X rays at the higher voltage.

placed on the tube's output window to enhance this effect. The maximum tube voltage determines maximum electron energy [expressed in kiloelectron volts (keV]. (Hence, the usage of kV peak to describe X-ray techniques.) The tungsten K-characteristic spectrum is seen when more than 69.52 kVp is applied to the X-ray tube.

INTERACTIONS OF X RAYS AND MATTER

Don't panic! This formula actually compresses most of the previous material in this chapter into one line (see Fig. 3-6). For now, we will assume that the absorber is a single element (e.g., carbon, iodine) and that the beam is monochromatic These restrictions will be removed later in this chapter.

The formula for calculating X-ray attenuation is

$$I = I_0 e^{-\mu(E,Z)\rho t}$$

where $\mu(E,Z)$ is the mass attenuation coefficient, E is the photon energy, Z is the atomic number of the attenuator, ρ is the physical density of the attenuator, and t is the path length through the attenuator.

Most of the radiation in a diagnostic X-ray beam is absorbed by superficial layers of material. Figure 3-7 is a plot of the absorption of monochromatic X-rays by carbon. Note that more than 80% of 20-keV photons are absorbed by the top 2 cm of carbon.

ATTENUATION COEFFICIENT

The attenuation coefficient of a material, $\mu(E,Z)$, depends on X-ray photon energy and the atomic composition of the attenuator. Several physical pro-

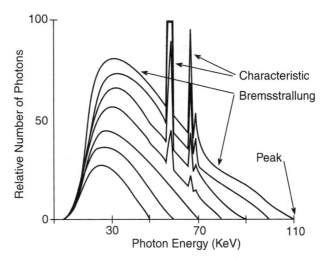

FIG. 3-5. X-ray spectra. Spectra of emitted X rays produced by a tungsten target when energized from 50 to 110 kVp. K-characteristic radiation is produced when the energizing voltage is above 69.52 kVp.

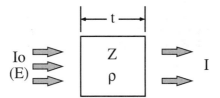

FIG. 3-6. Schematic X-ray interaction.

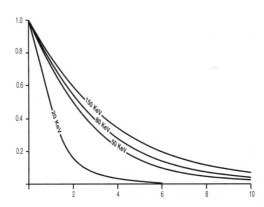

FIG. 3-7. Exponential attenuation of monochromatic radiation. By carbon at 20, 50, 80, and 150 keV. Note that lower energy photons are more rapidly attenuated.

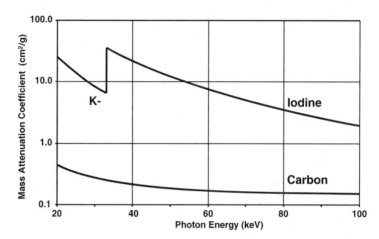

FIG. 3-8. Mass attenuation coefficients. For iodine and carbon as a function of photon energy. Note the logarithmic ordinate.

cesses occur at different energy ranges. The two of importance for diagnostic imaging are the photoelectric and Compton processes. Figure 3-8 illustrates the linear attenuation coefficient for carbon and iodine over the diagnostic imaging energy range. The attenuation of carbon is almost totally determined by the Compton process. The attenuation of iodine is the sum of these two processes. Photoelectric attenuation dominates at low energies, and Compton interactions dominate at high energies.

Photoelectric Process

The photoelectric process occurs when a photon interacts with an orbital electron of an atom. This process is most likely to occur if the incoming photon contains just a little more energy than the binding energy of the interacting electron. Iodine exhibits a K edge at exactly 33.2 keV (Fig. 3-4). A photoelectric interaction with a particular electron level cannot occur if the incoming photon's energy is less than the binding energy of that level. The K orbital electrons of participate in the photoelectric process for photons with energies above the binding energy. The probability of a photoelectric event decreases rapidly as photon energy increases. Because of the K edge, iodine is a much better X-ray absorber at 34 keV than it is at 33 keV. The K edge of carbon is 283 eV. Carbon does not exhibit significant photoelectric attenuation for diagnostic X rays.

The products of a photoelectric interaction are a fluorescence photon and the ejected electron. The kinetic energy of the ejected electron is the difference between the energy of the incoming photon and the binding energy of the electron. The electron's energy is dissipated close to the point of primary interaction. The energy of the fluorescence photon is the difference between the binding energy of the orbital electron and that of the lower energy electron that replaces it. Fluorescent photons are emitted isotropically (equal probability for any direction) from the atom. This fluorescence photon may travel some distance before it interacts with another atom.

Characteristic fluorescent-photon energies may be used to determine the composition of a sample.

Compton Effect

The Compton effect describes the interaction of an X-ray photon with an unbound electron. This condition is fulfilled if the photon's energy is much greater than the electron's binding energy. The probability of a Compton interaction declines slowly with increasing photon energy. The Compton effect is the main interaction process for diagnostic X rays in soft tissue. It is of increasing importance for iodine at energies significantly above iodine's K edge.

The products of a Compton interaction are a scattered X ray and a recoil electron. Some of the incident photon's energy is carried away from the interaction by the recoil electron. This energy is dissipated locally. The scattered photon contains the portion of the energy in the incoming photon not transferred to the electron. For diagnostic X rays, the scattered photon carries most of the incident photon's energy. In addition, in this energy range, scattered photons are emitted isotropically from the region of interaction. Most of the stray radiation in the laboratory is due to Compton interactions with the patient's tissues.

COMPOUND MATERIALS

Tissue is composed of different elements, and the X-ray beam is polychromatic. Both of these factors affect X-ray attenuation. Appendix A lists the mass attenuation coefficients of representative materials as a function of photon energy. Linear attenuation coefficients are obtained by multiplying the mass attenuation coefficient by density. The attenuation of a polychromatic beam is obtained by combining the monochromatic attenuation coefficients with the spectrum of the incident X-ray beam.

Note the similarity of the mass attenuation coefficients of muscle, water, and air over the entire energy range. This is why water is a good surrogate for muscle in phantoms and why measuring air dose tracks soft tissue dose.

THE EFFECT OF TUBE VOLTAGE ON CONTRAST

The attenuation coefficients of all of the materials decline with increasing photon energy (Appendix A). For now, photoelectric absorption edges are neglected. Subject contrast decreases as the attenuation coefficients decrease. This is true for differences in thickness and physical density. It is especially true for differences in atomic number (Z). This is because the mass attenuation coefficients of all the materials converge as photon energy increases. This can be seen in Appendix A by noting that the mass attenuation coefficients of water and iodine are 0.81 vs. 25.4 and 0.17 vs. 1.91 at 20 and 100 keV, respectively.

Why not use the lowest possible kVp and obtain the highest possible subject contrast? The electrical energy consumed by an X-ray tube is proportional to kVp. Efficiency of X-ray production is proportional to kVp^2. Because of the variation of absorption coefficient with energy, the intensity of radiation transmitted through a patient is proportional to $kVp^{4 \text{ to } 5}$. Imaging at high kVp minimizes the electrical load on the system and the radiation load on the patient. Controlling kVp is a key element in most feedback circuits. However, the contrast between iodine and tissue decreases as kVp increases. The visibility of vessels will therefore decrease with increasing voltage.

Iodine visibility decreases in thick patients because a higher kV is needed to "push" enough of the beam through the patient. This larger irradiated volume generates more scatter.

BEAM FILTRATION

The spectrum of photons produced by an X-ray tube includes energies ranging from a defined maximum (determined by the peak voltage applied to the tube) to a less well-defined minimum. The X-ray tube's anode and window absorb low energy (soft) radiation. Because soft radiation is also easily absorbed by tissue, it contributes to the patient's skin dose without contributing to image formation.

Aluminum has an appreciable photoelectric absorption coefficient at low energies. As in other materials, the attenuation coefficient of aluminum decreases with energy. Placing an aluminum filter on the output port of the X-ray tube reduces fluoroscopic patient dose by preferentially absorbing low-energy photons. This process is called "hardening the beam." This is seen in Figure 3-9.

The "quality" of an X-ray beam can be defined by its half-value layer (HVL). The HVL of a beam is the amount of material needed to reduce the beam's intensity by a factor of two. The physical properties of the absorber and the spectrum of the incident X-ray beam determine the HVL.

All of the HVLs of a monochromatic beam are identical (Fig. 3-10). This is not true for the polychromatic beam emerging from an X-ray tube. The first

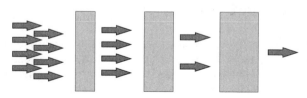

FIG. 3-9. Beam filtration. The aluminum filter hardens the beam by preferentially absorbing low-energy photons.

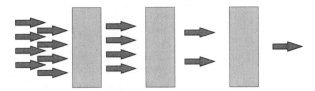

FIG. **3-10**. **Monochromatic beam.** Each of these equal thickness attenuators reduces the beam intensity by a factor of two.

HVL of a typical polychromatic fluoroscopic beam is around 3 mm of aluminum or 4 cm of tissue. HVL increases with increasing filtration and X-ray tube voltage. (The K-edge filters used for mammography are an important exception to this rule.) Figure 3-11 illustrates the increase in HVL with filtration.

The required minimum HVL for a diagnostic system increases with kVp. The requisite values are tabulated in the FDA's regulations. Compliance with these regulations ensures that the nonpenetrating radiation falling on the patient's skin is held to an acceptable minimum. Verification of minimum HVL is mandatory. Increasing beam hardness increases penetration of the beam through the patient. This means that less radiation needs to enter the patient to produce a constant exit dose (Fig. 3-12). Thus, harder beams reduce patient entrance dose.

Most interventional systems substantially exceed minimum values of HVL. Filtration between the X-ray tube and patient also absorbs some of the image-forming photon energies. Under most circumstances, adding excessive filtration further reductions in skin dose at the cost of a disproportionate increase in X-ray tube loading and an undesirable decrease in subject contrast. The resulting harder spectrum has more of its energy away from the iodine K-edge. This reduces iodine contrast. In addition, the effective output of the tube is reduced. When this happens, the imaging system often increases kVp. This further reduces contrast.

There are two exceptions to this rule: A thin (approximately 50 μm) copper filter is an important addition for interventional neuroradiology. Some newer systems use combinations of high-power X-ray tubes, copper filters, and special system-regulation-curves to better optimize the balance between patient dose and iodine contrast.

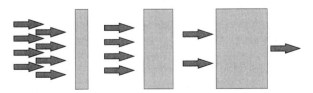

FIG. **3-11**. **Polychromatic beam.** The half value layer of a polychromatic beam increases as the beam is hardened.

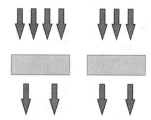

FIG. 3-12. Beam hardening. The HVL of the beam on the right is greater than the beam on the left. Less patient input dose is required on the right to produce the required output.

MINI COURSE

X-ray output is controlled by kVp, mA, and exposure time(s).

X-ray attenuation is dependent on the thickness, density, and atomic number of the absorber as well as by the X-ray beam spectrum.

Simply adding filtration to a beam decreases the patient's skin dose and the contrast of structures in the image.

SECTION TWO

Fluoroscopic Systems

4

X-Ray Generation and Control

REQUIREMENTS

X rays are produced when high-energy electrons interact with matter. This occurs in an X-ray tube. The purpose of the X-ray generator and its controls is to convert available electrical power into the precise form needed to operate the X-ray tube. In its simplest form (Fig. 4-1), the X-ray generator applies a high voltage, ranging from 50 to 150 peak kilovolts (kVp), which drives a direct current (mA) across the X-ray tube for a specific time(s). Another major circuit regulates the current flowing through the tube (mA). Radiation passing through the patient is measured by feedback circuits. This feedback signal is used to regulate the output of the generator in response to changes in patient size and position.

X-RAY GENERATORS

Generator Construction

The generator draws its energy from utility power lines. Input voltage is typically in the range from 110 to 440 V. This is usually supplied as three-phase AC at 60 Hz. Hospital wiring for X-ray generators needs some special attention. The minimum acceptable power rating of an interventional radiographic generator is 50 kW. To get an impression of the magnitude of this power level, a heavy-duty hair dryer uses about 1 kW.

> *Isolated generator power lines protect the remainder of the hospital from voltage transients caused by radiographic exposures.*

Less power is needed to supply mobile fluoroscopic generators such as those found in the operating room. Fluoroscopic performance of such systems is quite acceptable. Their radiographic capabilities are significantly below that of fixed installations.

43

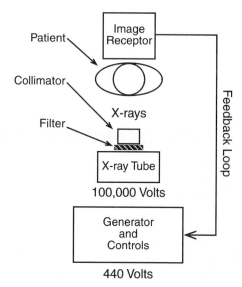

FIG. 4-1. Block diagram of an X-ray imaging system. The signal received by the image receptor is used to control generator output.

Mobile systems used for bedside radiography may derive their energy from onboard batteries. The batteries store enough energy to drive the system around the hospital and produce the relatively small number of radiographs acquired between recharges.

The X-ray tube voltages needed for proper imaging range from 50,000 to 150,000 V (50–150 kV). Ideally, the tube receives a constant (nonfluctuating or DC) voltage during the exposure.

Modern generators (Fig. 4-2) start their task by converting the energy flow to DC. This is done for engineering reasons. This energy drives a power oscillator. These oscillators are operated in the 500- to 5,000-Hz range. The operating sound made by the generator tells you its frequency. Audio frequencies permit the use of smaller high-voltage transformers than those required at the power line frequency of 60 Hz.

Rectifiers are placed between the output of the high-voltage transformer and the X-ray tube. These devices convert the transformer's AC output into the DC required by the X-ray tube.

X-ray tube current is determined by the temperature of the tube's filament. Electrons are emitted from a hot filament by the process of thermionic emission. Those circuits needed to set the filament temperature and thereby control the current flowing through the X-ray tube (mA). These circuits are not explicitly shown in the diagram.

The high-voltage transformers, rectifiers, and other elements are placed in a "high-voltage" tank. The outer electrical layer of the tank, high-voltage cables, and X-ray tube are connected to ground. This is a necessary protection against electrical shock.

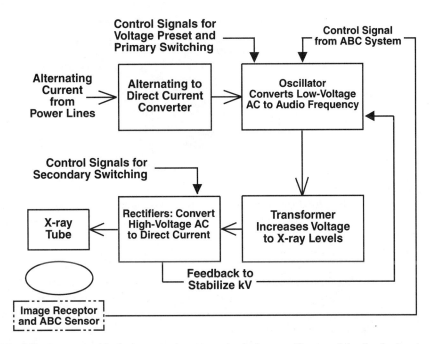

FIG. 4-2. Generator block diagram showing principal power flows and feedback circuits. (Please refer to the text for an explanation.)

The time of X-ray production is controlled by applying and removing power to the X-ray tube. This is done using electronic switches in the oscillator, high-voltage tank, or by the use of a grid in the X-ray tube.

Electronic control of the oscillator determines the voltage applied to the X-ray tube. Control signals are supplied by the system controller, high-voltage tank, and automatic brightness control system (ABC). The system-controller signals establish the initial operating factors.

Instruments in the high-voltage tank monitor kV and mA. Signals from these instruments are used in feedback circuits to maintain required operating conditions.

The multitude of sensors and feedback controls provides "closed loop" control of all critical operating parameters. These components provide stable long-term system performance. The intervals needed between routine calibrations can be safely extended relative to previous generations of "open loop" systems. Of course, maintenance, quality control measurements, and calibration are needed when "smoke" comes out of the system or an X-ray tube or other major component is replaced.

Automatic Brightness Control (ABC)

Feedback circuits to control the generator measure the intensity of the light emitted from a portion of the image intensifier. The net result is maintenance of constant image brightness over a range of patient thickness. Control is obtained by adjusting the X-ray output of the system. This circuit is often

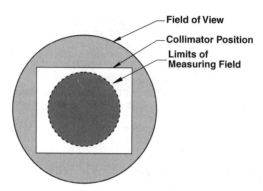

FIG. 4-3. ABC measuring field. A typical ABC system measures the peak or average brightness of the portion of the image inside the measuring field. Here, the X-ray beam totally illuminates the measuring field.

called an automatic brightness control (ABC). Fig. 4-3 sketches a typical ABC measuring field. The dotted circle indicates the extent of the measuring field. Such measuring fields are typically 40–80% of the diameter of the working field–of–view of the image intensifier.

Some systems take a simple average of the brightness in the measuring field. Other systems are designed to search for maximum brightness. All systems perform equally well when the X-ray field is larger than the measuring field and a relatively homogeneous portion of the patient.

Figure 4-4 illustrates combinations of measuring field and X-ray field sizes. Figure 4-4A shows both large X-ray and measuring fields. Such a combination provides a signal that represents the average transmission through a large portion of the patient's anatomy. In Figure 4-4B, the X-ray field has been collimated to less than the measuring field. The unirradiated portion of the measuring field lowers the average. This results is too much X-ray output (too bright an image), as the system attempts to image outside the collimators. A small measuring field is shown in Fig. 4-4, C and D. This produces the correct output if it overlies an average density tissue. It will produce too much output if the measuring field is over bone and insufficient output if the measuring field is over lung.

The relationships between measuring-field size, shape, and averaging technique are not confined to fluoroscopy. Similar considerations apply to measuring the brightness of photographic scenes. The ability to match a measuring technique to a particular task has improved with improvements in the ability to optically dissect the scene. Operator intervention may be needed to select the appropriate measuring program.

Exposure Time Control

The system is often switched on and off at the generator. The tube and generator are connected by high-voltage cables. These cables store electrical charge when voltage is applied. This charge continues to supply energy to the X-ray tube after the switch is opened. This will prolong the exposure time by

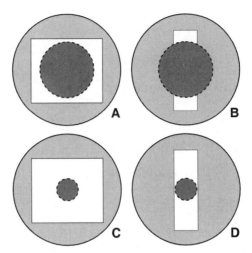

FIG. 4-4. **Relationships between measuring fields and X-ray fields.** A: Large measuring and X-ray fields average a large fraction of the patient's anatomy. B: Large measuring and small X-ray fields produce too low an average reading. (The unirradiated region contributes to the average.) C: A small measuring field averages only a small portion of the patient's anatomy. This can give a false reading if it is over lung or spine. D: A small measuring field minimizes the effect of measuring outside the X-ray field.

a certain amount. Cable discharge time is prolonged when the cables are long and the X-ray tube current is low. This can lead to excessive motion unsharpness. Some X-ray tubes employ a biased cathode to electrically switch the current on and off. For historical reasons, this is called "grid switching." When its operating parameters are compatible with the required radiographic technique, grid switching eliminates the problem of cable discharge.

THE X-RAY TUBE

The X-ray tube converts electrical energy into X-rays. Basic physical factors make this a very inefficient process. Less than 1% of the applied electrical energy is converted to X rays. The remaining 99% heats the tube's target. Tubes are constructed to handle this waste heat without damage. Much of the aggravation about system-imposed delays is due to the time needed for heat management. Modern tubes are capable of handling several times as much heat as those of the early 1990s. These tubes can deliver significantly more radiation without overload than was possible a decade or so ago.

The essential elements of a medium power X-ray tube are shown in Figure 4-5. The vacuum tube, stator, and cooling components are contained in a protective housing (Fig. 4-6). Oil filling contributes to the system's electrical insulation as well as participating in the tube's heat management process.

The housing protects patients and staff from electrical shock by providing a grounded outer shield. Lead absorbs radiation going in directions other than those intended to be the useful beam.

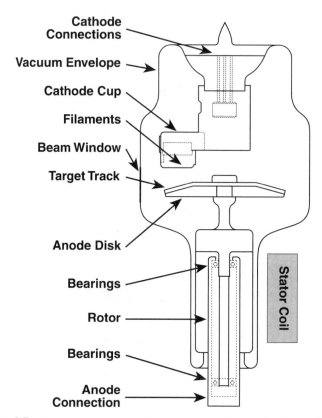

Cathode Connections

Vacuum Envelope

Cathode Cup

Filaments

Beam Window

Target Track

Anode Disk

Bearings

Rotor

Bearings

Anode Connection

Stator Coil

FIG. 4-5. Components of a medium-power rotating anode X-ray tube.

The tube's vacuum envelope provides the necessary high-vacuum environ-ment for the remaining components. Many vacuum envelopes are made of metal instead of glass.

Electrons are generated in the hot filament by the process of thermionic emission. Tube current is controlled by adjusting the filament temperature. This can take a few seconds because this is a thermal process. As previously indicated, elements in the tube current circuit provide the feedback needed to stabilize the tube current. Filaments are maintained at a lower standby tem-perature unless a radiographic exposure is in progress. This is an important factor in tube life.

The electrons that constitute the tube current (mA) are electrostatically directed to the focal spot by the cathode cup. Most X-ray tubes have two differently sized filaments in two cathode cups. Heating the appropriate fila-ment determines whether the large or small focal spot is active (Fig. 4-7).

The target of most X-ray tubes is tungsten. The combination of high melt-ing point (3400°C) and high atomic number (74) makes this the best choice for most situations. A small percentage of rhenium is usually alloyed with the tungsten to maintain the smoothness of the target. This alloy provides a more consistent X-ray output over the tube's life. The body of the anode is often

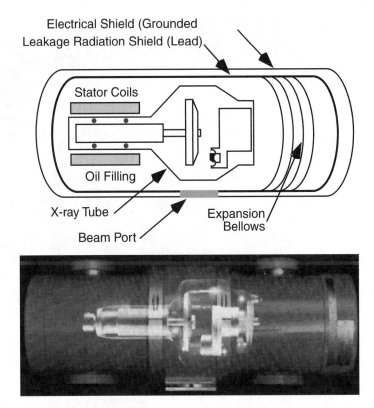

Electrical Shield (Grounded
Leakage Radiation Shield (Lead)

Stator Coils

Oil Filling

X-ray Tube

Beam Port

Expansion
Bellows

FIG. 4-6. **X-ray tube in its protective housing.** The insulating oil expands as it is heated. An internal switch disables the system when the bellows overexpand. [Photograph courtesy of Philips Medical Systems.]

made of molybdenum or graphite. These materials provide good thermal conductivity and large heat storage capability.

Electrical and thermal safety circuits limit X-ray tube operation to protect tube elements from thermal damage.

Even tungsten does not always stand up to the rigors of high-power radiography without melting. Several techniques are used to spread the energy in the electron beam over enough target material to avoid meltdowns shown, for example, in Figure 4-8.

The first method of spreading out the beam is called the line-focus-principle. In Figure 4-9, the central ray of the X-ray beam is perpendicular to the electron stream. The focal spot on the anode is at an angle to the central ray. Decreasing this angle produces the same square effective focal spot using a larger rectangular physical focus. This increases the tube rating. There is a price to be paid. Decreasing the anode angle decreases the maximum available size of the X-ray field. In addition, X-ray fields produced by smaller angle anodes are less homogeneous than those produced by larger angle anodes. This is called the heel effect. Nonuniformity may be an important factor in video-densitometric analysis.

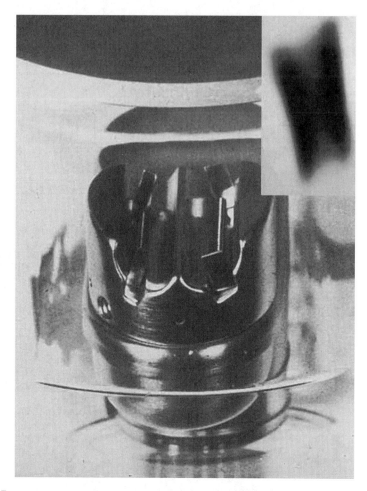

FIG. 4-7. Cathode assembly with filaments for large and small focal spots. The insert in the upper right is a pinhole photograph of an actual focal spot. Note the relative nonuniformity. (This focal spot is well within industry specifications.)

Most tubes incorporate a rotating anode. Moving "cool" target material through the electron beam enables much higher power levels than possible with a stationary anode. Increasing the anode's diameter increases the track length and therefore the short-term tube ratings (Fig. 4-10). The larger diameter anode is heavier. Such an anode is harder to start and stop and places greater stress on the bearings. A benefit of the larger anode is an increase in anode heat-storage capacity. This is attributable to its greater mass. Interventional systems usually incorporate tubes with large anode diameters.

Anode rotation is accomplished by electromagnetically linking motive power from a stator coil located outside the vacuum envelope to a rotor coil located on the anode's shaft. Typical operating speeds range from 3000 to −10,000 rpm.

Support of the rotor is a critical design element. Conventional tubes use ball bearings. The anode in such tubes is usually at a stop during fluoroscopy.

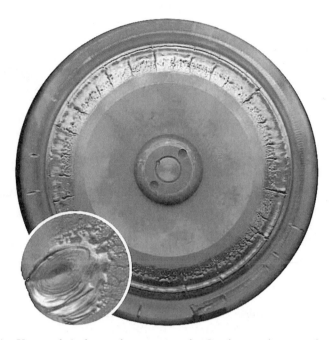

FIG. 4-8. An X-ray tube's damaged rotating anode. Overheating has caused various types of damage. The insert on the lower left is a magnified view of a stationary melt on the anode.

It must be rapidly brought up to operating speed before initiating a radiographic exposure. Acceleration time is one of the reasons for the few seconds of delay required between fluoroscopy and radiography. Electromagnetic brakes are applied to the rotor after a run.

Anode stem and bearing design is interesting. The bearings have to function with anodes ranging from room temperature up to white heat. They must provide a path to conduct the X-ray tube current. Bearings cannot be lubricated with any substance that could contaminate the vacuum. Lead and silver

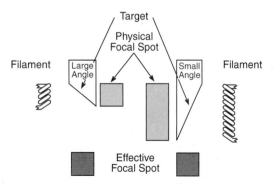

FIG. 4-9. Line focus principle. The increased foreshortening produced by a small anode angle permits a larger physical focus for the same effective focal spot size.

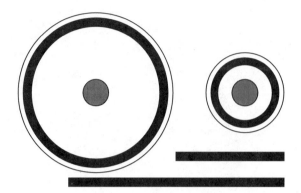

FIG. 4-10. Focal track length. The track length is proportional to the diameter of the anode disk. The mass of a uniform thickness anode is proportional to the square of the diameter. The larger diameter anode will also have a larger heat storage capacity.

alloy balls have the necessary properties. Certain newer tube types use liquid metal bearings. The anodes of these tubes are brought up to operating speed when the system is turned on in the morning. The anodes remain spinning all day with no loss of tube life.

Heat from the focal track flows into the body of the anode. This takes a fraction of a second. Sufficient time must be allowed for heat flow. Figure 4-11 illustrates the single exposure target ratings for the small focus of a typical angiographic tube. Exceeding these ratings, or other tube ratings, can cause damage. The combination of low rotation speed and high loading caused the tungsten to melt on the anode, as shown in Figure 4-8. Several minutes are

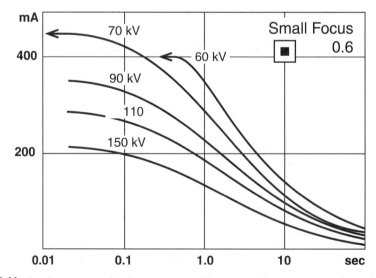

FIG. 4-11. Single exposure focal spot ratings. The ratings for any given voltage decrease as the exposure time is increased because of increasing target temperature. Specialized tables are used to determine safe ratings for rapid sequence exposures.

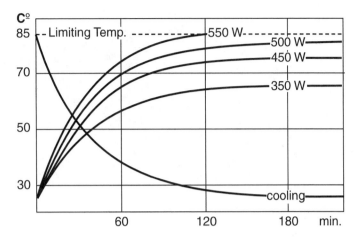

FIG. 4-12. Housing cooling curves. Too high an average power level can bring this housing to its limiting temperature in a short time. The overheated housing will take hours to return to room temperature.

needed for heat to flow from the anode to the tube housing. Several tens of minutes are needed to move heat energy from the housing to the environment (Fig. 4-12). In the absence of a cooling system, hours are needed until an overheated housing returns to room temperature. Forced cooling systems are available and should be used in angiographic situations.

X-RAY BEAM COLLIMATORS

> Minimizing field size (by collimating the beam) is a rare example of a simultaneous improvement in image quality and a decrease of radiation risk.

X rays are emitted isotropically from the focal spot. A port in the lead shielded tube housing defines the maximum size of the X-ray beam. Tube ports are manufactured to fully irradiate the largest image receptor at the shortest working distance (Fig. 4-13). In most circumstances, the uncollimated beam is larger than the image receptor. This is undesirable from both image quality and radiation protection points of view.

One should only use radiation in amounts that benefit the patient. Using an X-ray beam that is much larger than the image receptor is wasteful of radiation and produces unnecessary risk. Subject contrast is maximized and radiation risk to both patient and staff is minimized by collimating the X-ray beam.

The amount of scattered radiation produced in the patient increases with field size. Increased scatter decreases image contrast. Staff and patient radiation risks also increase with beam size. Adjustable collimators are provided to limit the radiation beam to at least the size of the active image receptor and, ideally, to the size of the region of immediate clinical interest.

As shown in Figure 4-14, there are several ways of collimating an X-ray beam. In Figure 4-14A, collimation is accomplished by means of a simple

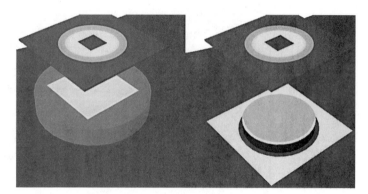

FIG. 4-13. **An aperture plate limits the emitted beam size.** The beam is confined when the image receptor is close to the X-ray tube (*left*) and is too large when the same image receptor is far from the X-ray tube (*right*).

aperture plate. This works well enough to manage the radiation emerging from the focal spot. However, X-ray tubes produce a significant amount of off-focus radiation. Such radiation is produced when electrons are scattered inside the X-ray tube and eventually produce X-rays by interacting elsewhere in the tube. Off-focus radiation can be reduced by introducing a second aperture (Fig. 4-14B). It is further reduced by minimizing the size of the aperture located at the X-ray tube port (Fig. 4-14C). These reductions increase the effective radiographic contrast of the image.

Collimators can be either fixed or variable. Fixed collimators have no place in modern interventional systems. Variable collimators are required to self-adapt to changes in the image receptor's field of view and to changes in the source-to-image-receptor distance (SID). (Further information about collimators may be found in Chapter 13.)

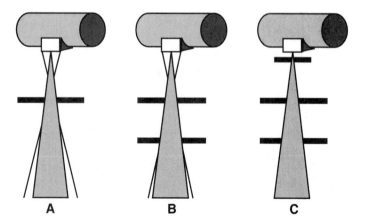

FIG. 4-14. **Collimation.** A: Single aperture plate defines field size. It passes significant off-focus radiation. B: Double bladed collimator reduces off-focus radiation. C: Additional aperture near the X-ray tube provides further reduction of off-focus radiation.

MINI COURSE

Image intensity measurements and closed-loop control circuits provide consistent imaging performance.

Almost all of the electrical energy applied to an X-ray tube is converted into heat. Tube design is focused on safely handling this heat.

Collimators control the size and shape of the X-ray beam. One should never irradiate objects that are not within the active field-of view of the image receptor.

5

X-Ray Image Receptors
(The Image Intensifier)

Fluorescence is the physical process that converts X-ray energy into visible light. The two main steps are the absorption of an X-ray photon by a phosphor crystal and the subsequent emission of many visible-light photons from the crystal. A modern fluoroscopic screen detects more than half of the incident X rays. A single X-ray photon contains between 20 and 150 kiloelectron volts (keV) of energy. Light photons contain around 3 eV. Thus, a single X-ray photon can theoretically produce tens of thousands of light photons. Most fluorescent phosphors actually produce about a thousand light photons for each detected X-ray photon.

In former times, simple fluoroscopic screens were used at reasonable dose levels. This required that the operator be fully adapted to the dark. Direct fluoroscopy is no longer permitted in much of the world.

DARK ADAPTATION

The dark-adapted eye is a sensitive light detector. Full dark adaptation takes about 30 min (Fig. 5-1). Perhaps some readers will recall physicians dark adapted by wearing red goggles. Screen fluoroscopy required working in a dark room. The dark procedure room does not particularly enhance the efficiency of support staff or promote patient comfort. Dark adaptation also reduces both the spatial and temporal sensitivity of the eye (Figs. 5-2 and 5-3).

Increasing the brightness of the image delivered to the observer by at least 1000 times (hopefully without increasing dose) eliminates the need for dark adaptation. The first X-ray image intensifiers meeting this requirement appeared in medical practice in the late 1950s. Early systems provided a direct optical image. These devices also produced enough light to expose the film in a cinefluorographic camera. The latter is a critical technical prerequisite for cardiac angiography.

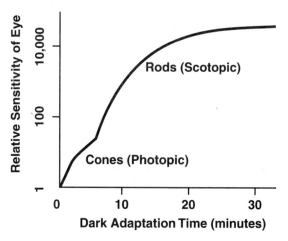

FIG. 5-1. Dark adaptation. Increases the sensitivity of the eye by several orders of magnitude. Causes a loss in visual acuity when going from cone (bright) to rod (dim) vision (see Figs. 5-2 and 5-3).

Closed circuit television systems replaced direct viewing in the 1960s. A variety of electronic means began to displace optical cine-film recording in the late 1980s. The direct X-ray-to-digital converter is likely to phase out the image intensifier tube itself in the early 21st century.

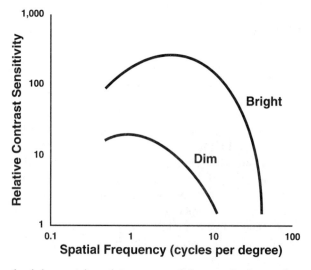

FIG. 5-2. Sketch of the spatial resolving power of the eye. Cycles per degree can be converted into line pairs per millimeter when the viewing distance is known.

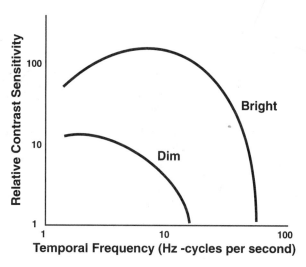

FIG. 5-3. **Sketch of the temporal resolving power of the eye.** This sketch does not include the effects of flicker.

IMAGE INTENSIFIER ANATOMY

Figure 5-4 is a schematic sagittal section of a single-mode X-ray image intensifier. Figure 5-5 illustrates the sequence of energy conversion steps that occur within the image intensifier.

The active elements of the tube are in a vacuum. The X-ray beam enters the tube through an input window. This window must simultaneously be strong enough to withstand atmospheric pressure and thin enough to minimize the attenuation of the input X-ray beam.

The input screen or input phosphor is composed of cesium iodide (CsI). The screen is manufactured by growing CsI crystals as a layer of "needles" on a thin glass substrate. The fluorescence process converts the incident X-ray signal into a visible light image. Each detected X-ray photon produces about a thousand light photons. The CsI "needle" structure acts as a light pipe. This minimizes lateral light diffusion and results in improved spatial resolution.

Thicker CsI layers are better X-ray absorbers than thinner layers. However, because the light piping is not perfect, there is more light diffusion in thicker layers. A typical 0.2-mm-thick layer absorbs more than half of the incident X-ray beam. This is a reasonable tradeoff between dose efficiency and spatial resolution.

The photocathode is coated on the other side of the input-screen substrate. The glass is a barrier between the chemically incompatible CsI and photocathode. The photocathode absorbs light photons emerging from the input screen. This results in the emission of photoelectrons. In the optical photoelectric process, the energy of a single absorbed light photon ejects a single electron from the photocathode. Competing processes absorb light without the emission of photoelectrons. The principal cause of image intensifier degradation is a chemical change in the photocathode over time. This reduces the

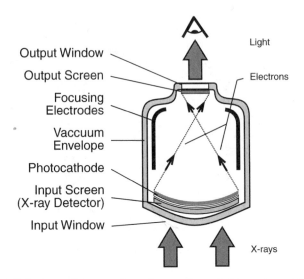

FIG. 5-4. Sagittal section through a single-mode image intensifier.

number of photoelectrons produced for a given number of incident light photons.

Photoelectrons emerge from the photocathode with very little kinetic energy. Indeed, ideal focusing occurs when the fresh photoelectrons have zero energy. A series of electrodes accelerate the photoelectrons to a typical energy of 40 keV. It also focuses them onto a smaller output screen. These two effects separately contribute to the image intensifier brightness gain.

The output screen is a ZnCdS layer. The energy carried by the electrons produces light by the fluorescence process. (ZnCdS was also the phosphor used in direct fluoroscopic screens.) The energy carried by each electron produces thousands of fluorescent light photons. This light emerges from the image intensifier through an output window.

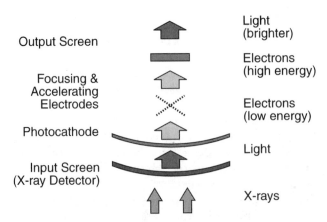

FIG. 5-5. Energy conversion steps in a single-mode X-ray image intensifier.

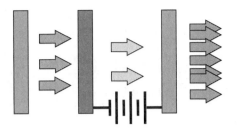

FIG. 5-6. Electronic brightness gain. Electrons emitted by the photocathode gain energy from an electric field. These electrons cause an output screen to fluoresce. Many light photons emerge from the output screen for each light photon entering the photocathode.

ZnCdS produces green fluorescent light matching the peak spectral sensitivity of the dark-adapted eye. This green output was needed for direct fluoroscopy and early image intensifiers.

Electronic brightness gain (Fig. 5-6) occurs because the voltage applied to the image intensifier electrodes (40 kV) supplies energy to each photoelectron as it travels from photocathode to output screen. Light photons produced in the input screen have energies of a few electron volts. Thus, a single 40-keV electron has enough energy to produce thousands of light photons in the output screen. Military low-light-level goggles use only use electronic brightness gain.

Minification brightness gain (Fig. 5-7) occurs when the output image is smaller than the input image. Minification gain (G_m) is proportional to the ratio of the areas of the input and output screens:

$$G_m = \text{input screen area/output screen area}$$

For example, G_m is calculated for 9- and 5-in. input screens with a constant 1-in. output screen:

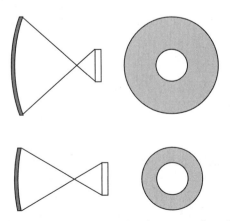

FIG. 5-7. Minification brightness gain. All of the electrons collected from a large area on the input structure converge on the smaller output screen. Minification gain is proportional to the ratio of these two areas.

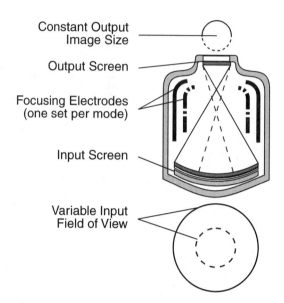

FIG. 5-8. Dual-mode image intensifier. Two sets of electrodes focus a larger or smaller portion of the input structure onto the fixed size output screen. There is less minification gain in the smaller FOV (zoomed mode). Additional electrodes enable additional zoom modes.

$$G_m (9) = (\pi 9^2/4)/(\pi 1^2/4) = 9^2/1^2 = (9/1)^2 = 81$$

$$G_m (5) = (\pi 5^2/4)/(\pi 1^2/4) = 5^2/1^2 = (4/1)^2 = 25$$

Multimode image intensifiers contain several sets of electrodes within the vacuum container (Fig. 5-8). Selecting electrodes that focus a smaller part of the input screen onto the output screen magnifies the image. A magnified (zoom) mode has less minification gain. The equations given above are as applicable to the individual modes of a 9/5 dual-mode image intensifier as they are to separate single mode tubes. One consequence is an increase in patient skin dose rate when the image is zoomed.

IMAGE INTENSIFIER PERFORMANCE

Conversion Factor

The amplification of an image intensifier was originally described in terms of its brightness gain relative to a directly exposed fluoroscopic screen. Conversion factor (G_x) is a more objective measure of performance. This international unit is a measure of the amount of light produced by the tube for a given X-ray input.

The conversion factor of the smaller field of view (magnification mode) of a dual-mode image intensifier is less than the G_x of the larger field of view (Fig. 5-9). Electronically imaging a smaller portion of the input screen onto

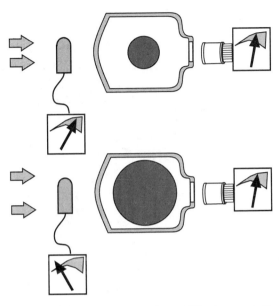

FIG. 5-9. **Effect of zoom mode on conversion factor.** The lesser minification gain in the magnified mode reduces G_X. More radiation maintains image brightness.

the fixed size output screen magnifies the image. As noted above, this maneuver reduces minification gain. Imaging systems must produce the constant light output needed by the cameras. Thus, magnification modes require higher image intensifier dose levels than nonmagnification modes.

There are some interesting clinical and dosimetric implications. Simple calculations will show that the dose area product (DAP) is essentially independent of zoom mode for constant light output. Patient skin dose increases as image intensifier entrance dose increases. The exact relationship depends on the engineering details of any given imaging system. The cost of using high-magnification factors during long interventional procedures is the increased probability of crossing the deterministic threshold and inflicting patient skin damage. It should be noted that a DAP instrument will not directly warn the operator about this increased risk.

Selecting a nonmagnified mode places less of a load on the generator and tube.

The effect is different when the X-ray beam collimates within the selected field–of–view (FOV). As shown in Figure 5-10, the image does not fill the output screen. The ratio of the areas of the input and output images is a constant. The conversion factor and therefore the image intensifier entrance dose remain the same. DAP decreases because of decreased beam size. This decreases the total amount of scatter produced in the patient. This yields better image contrast and less stochastic risk to both patient and staff.

The down side of using collimation instead of zoom is a smaller image and perhaps less spatial resolution. Some modern fluoroscopes provide digital zoom. The image processor digitally magnifies the image to fill the monitor. The actual spatial resolution is unchanged. However, this technique may increase

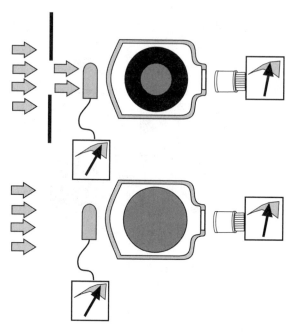

FIG. 5-10. **Effect of collimation on conversion factor.** G_X is constant for a given mode. The output image is smaller for a collimated beam. Radiation requirements are constant.

the operator's ability to see details in the image if magnified structures now appear with a size closer to the peak spatial sensitivity of the eye (Fig. 5-2).

A word of caution is applicable to image intensifier magnification mode and digital zoom: Live fluoroscopy or fluorography without the X-ray collimator following the zoom mode is illegal and can be dangerous. It is simply not appropriate to irradiate substantial volumes of nonimaged tissue.

Modulation Transfer Function

A modulation transfer function (MTF) curve can be used to display imaging performance. Figure 5-11 is a sketch of the MTF curve for a dual-mode image intensifier. This plot shows the ability to image objects of different sizes. MTF plots are in units of frequency (e.g., line pairs per millimeter). The lower set of targets indicates the meaning of spatial frequency. The contrast of the upper set of targets indicates the MTF at different spatial frequencies. (Figs. 5-2 and 5-3 are MTF plots for the spatial and temporal response of the eye.)

The image intensifier's ability to fully reproduce the modulation of even the largest objects is not perfect. The physical cause is the presence of diffuse light inside the image intensifier. Causes include absorption of radiation by structures other than the input screen, scattering of electrons by residual gas molecules, and light diffusion in the screens. This is shown as the dip in the MTF curve at low frequencies. Modern tubes have low-frequency MTF values above 95%.

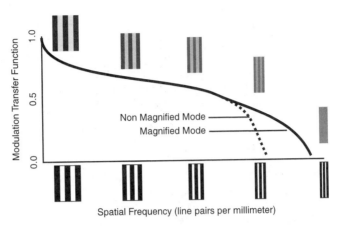

FIG. 5-11. MTF curve for a dual-mode image intensifier. The bar patterns above the curve are an impression of the contrast at different spatial frequencies. Note that the nonmagnified mode has less limiting resolution than the magnified mode.

The ability to precisely focus the electron image and the structure of the output-screen limit the visualization of tiny objects (high spatial frequencies). Imaging a smaller area of patient on the fixed output window can improve spatial resolution. The MTF of the nonmagnified mode cuts off at frequencies lower than those of the magnified mode. The MTF plot of this tube tells us that the magnified mode will allow the visualization of objects smaller than the nonmagnified mode will allow.

Actual performance will also depend on many other imaging-system elements. The image intensifier tube is only one component in the imaging chain. The overall system MTF involves additional factors. These include geometric and motion unsharpness and the MTF of the television system.

Optimum system MTF differs for different imaging tasks.

Image Nonuniformities

The electro-optical design of the image intensifier tube requires the photocathode to be on a spherical surface. This is why the field of view is circular. Focusing a curved input screen onto a flat output screen produces pincushion distortion (Fig. 5-12). Magnetic fields, including the Earth's natural magnetic field, disturb electrostatic focusing and thereby induce further spatial distortions in the image. In extreme cases, residual magnetism in a structural steel of a building can render a room unsuitable for fluoroscopy. There are more distortions in larger FOV modes than in smaller FOV modes. The distorted image of a uniform mesh is well known. Some analytic software corrects for this effect.

The collection efficiency of the electro-optical focusing lenses in the image intensifier, and the optical lenses downstream in the system, is better toward the center than in the periphery (Fig. 5-13). This radial fall off in brightness is called vignetting.

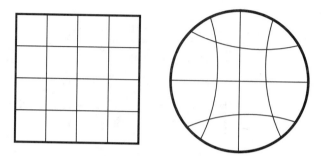

FIG. 5-12. Sketch of pincushion distortion. The curved input screen and stray magnetic fields distort the image of a square grid.

OPTICS

Transmitting the image from the intensifier to the observer's eye or to a camera requires an optical system. Figure 5-14 illustrates the essential elements of a single-channel optical system. The first (collimating) lens is focused on the output screen This collimating lens converts the image into a parallel light bundle. A second (focusing) lens delivers a focused image onto the camera. Fluoroscopic system lenses have very good light-collection efficiency (low minimum f number).

The parallel light bundle between the two lenses provides many technical benefits. The most important of these is the insertion of an optical diaphragm into this space. Setting the diaphragm opening controls the amount of light delivered to the camera.

Image intensifiers usually produce too much light for optimal image quality. The ultimate source of image noise should always be statistical fluctuations in the X-ray beam. Increasing dose (more precisely the amount of radiation detected by the image intensifier) reduces the percent fluctuation and hence the perceived noise. Figure 5-15 illustrates the transfer stages through the image intensifier. In most modern systems, the minimum number of carriers occurs at the X-ray detection stage. This stage is called the "quantum sink" of the system.

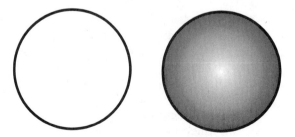

FIG. 5-13. Sketch of vignetting. Light collection efficiency is less toward the periphery of a lens than in the center. This produces the radial decrease in brightness (*right*).

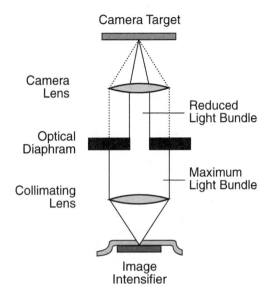

FIG. 5-14. Single-channel optical system. The collimating lens produces a parallel light bundle. Adjusting the optical diaphragm controls light intensity. The focusing lens converges the light bundle onto the camera.

It is possible to regulate image brightness by adjusting X-ray intensity and pass all available light to the observer. The conversion factor (G_X) of a new tube is usually so high that this produces an unacceptably noisy image. Closing the aperture of the optical diaphragm reduces the number of light photons delivered to the camera for each detected X-ray photon. Image noise is decreased when system control elements compensate for this loss of light by increasing X-ray dose.

As the image intensifier ages, its photocathode becomes less efficient. Each incident X-ray photon produces fewer light photons. Opening the optical di-

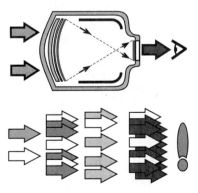

FIG. 5-15. Quantum sink. There are a finite number of information carriers at each stage of the image intensification process. Image noise is governed by the stage with the fewest number of carriers. This quantum sink is usually the X-ray detection stage.

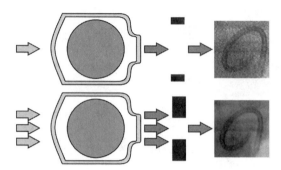

FIG. 5-16. **Regulating input dose and image noise.** When the optical diaphragm is open, few X-ray photons are needed to operate the camera. The image is noisy. Closing the diaphragm throws light away. Producing more X-rays reduces noise.

aphragm maintains camera brightness. Eventually, the diaphragm will be wide open. At this point, increasing X-ray intensity is the only available compensation for further image intensifier degradation. The image intensifier should be replaced before this occurs.

The optical diaphragm is an essential operational tool for clinically controlling image noise. As shown in Figure 5-16, a large diaphragm setting passes a large fraction of the image intensifier light to the camera. A small diaphragm setting allows only a small portion of the light to pass. More radiation is needed to meet the total light requirement of the camera. The additional radiation reduces statistical noise in the image. The two images shown in Figures 2-16 and 2-17 were acquired a few seconds apart by the same imaging system. Figure 2-16 was made with the dose from a single fluoroscopic frame. Figure 2-17 is the mask for a digital subtraction angiogram (DSA) run. Closing the diaphragm drove the system to deliver approximately 200 times as much radiation to the image intensifier.

It is convenient to view the image during film fluorography. Placing a partially silvered mirror (beam splitter) in the light bundle during cinefluorography divides the available light between the fluoroscopic television camera and the cine-film camera (Fig. 5-17).

To meet the more demanding image noise requirements for cinefluorography, as much radiation is needed for a single cine frame as for a second of fluoroscopy. There is a large amount of light available in the system. The few percent needed to operate the video camera does not substantially affect exposure of the cine film. (In most cases, there is so much light that secondary optical diaphragms in the cameras are needed to fine tune the system.)

The beam splitter is removed during fluoroscopy. All of the light goes to the television camera. Even when all of the light is used for fluoroscopy, the image appears noisier because fluoroscopic dose rates are lower (true if the quantum sink is the number of detected X-ray photons).

Digital cine systems reduce dose during fluoroscopy by opening the diaphragm and reduce noise by closing the diaphragm during cine acquisition. All other aspects of the imaging system are identical. Intermediate operating values are important in certain clinical situations.

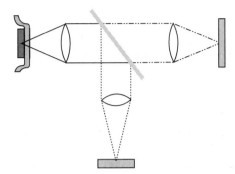

FIG. 5-17. **Two-channel beam splitter.** A partially silvered mirror diverts a fraction of the available light into a second camera port. Removing the mirror causes all of the light to enter the straight through port. The beam splitter is not found in a pure digital imaging system.

A LOOK BACK AND A LOOK AHEAD

The X-ray image intensifier was one of the technologies necessary for the development of coronary angiography in the 1950s. It enabled the operator to work with reasonable room illumination. It also provided sufficient light to expose photographic film. The introduction of CsI in the 1970s brought the quantum efficiency of the image intensifier to the 50% range. An ideal system can only reduce dose by a factor of two without increasing image noise. The structure of the CsI layer also resulted in a reduction of large-area–contrast loss and an improvement in MTF.

Image acquisition through a video chain into a digital image processor is an essential technology of the 1990s. Such systems free the operator from mechanical and chemical constraints inherent in film recording. Operating "digital" systems using the same X-ray spectra and frame rates as the predecessors does not save patient dose. However, other aspects of system setup and operation have also evolved.

There is a substantial net patient dose saving when one compares 1990 and 1998 systems from the same manufacturer in adjacent rooms. Some of this is attributable to modified X-ray spectra, another portion to a reduction in cine-frame rates from 30 to 15 frames per second (fps), and the remaining fraction to the operator's willingness to accept more noise.

The image intensifier described in this chapter is unlikely to survive beyond the first decade of the third millennium. Direct detection image receptors (perhaps less than 10 cm thick) are emerging. The limiting factor in their widespread introduction is the nontrivial industrial technology needed to reliably manufacture large defect free devices. The 14-in. screen on the laptop computer used to write this book is an example of a 1024×768 pixel transistor array that might be large enough for cardiovascular imaging. Prototype devices have been demonstrated using both a fluorescent-screen and a photo-pickup matrix or an array of X-ray-sensitive elements. Imaging characteristics partially depend on the number of active pixels in the selected FOV. Some inherent problems such as pincushion distortion, vingetting, and large-area–contrast loss should disappear. Flat receptors should be at least as dose efficient as the best conventional image intensifier. Stay tuned for future developments.

MINI COURSE

In a well-designed system, image noise is decreased by increasing image receptor input dose.

Increasing magnification by zooming an image intensifier usually requires an increase in dose.

Increasing the size of the optical diaphragm compensates for image intensifier deterioration (up to the point where the diaphragm is fully open).

6

Fluoroscopic and Fluorographic Cameras

Cameras and display devices transfer images from the image intensifier to the observer's eye. A variety of direct vision and photographic camera technologies were previously used (Fig. 6-1). The cinefluorographic camera is the last vestige of this era. Video-based systems are preferred at the start of the new millennium.

At the time of this writing, we are at the cusp of the transformation from "film" to "filmless" fluorography. This chapter includes a review of important aspects of the film era. Many of these concepts have direct counterparts in analog and digital video systems. Several previous technological constraints do not limit modern systems.

Video viewing and film recording were essential parts of the 1970–1990 systems. Broadcast television standards defined video technology. Most film formats and cameras derive from Hollywood. A third, and often ignored, leg of the technology tripod is the frequency of the AC power supplied by electric companies.

The standard power line frequency in the United States is 60 cycles per second (60 Hz). The European standard is 50 Hz. Broadcast video relies on the power line to provide synchronization between studio cameras and home receivers. Consequently, the standard video frame rate is 30 frames per second (fps) in the United States and 25 fps in Europe.

Angiographers are accustomed to viewing television images during cinefluorography. Image artifacts are avoided by filming at frame rates that are multiples or submultiples of the video frame rate. This is why medical cinefilm frame rates are 60 or 30 fps (50 or 25 fps in Europe).

QUALITY MOTION PICTURES

A sports fan watching a ball game sees players smoothly moving around a uniformly illuminated field. A moving picture should have the same visual

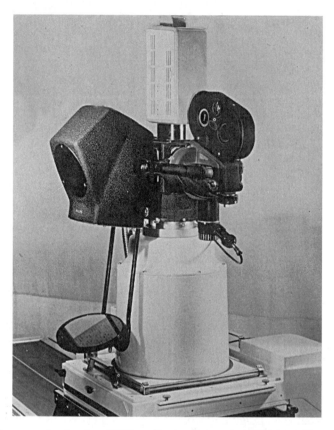

FIG. 6-1. An example of a circa 1970 cardiac imaging system. The cine-film camera is on the *right*, the video camera is on the top, and a mirror viewing system is on the *left*. Television was not reliable enough to do without the mirror. [Photo courtesy of Philips Medical Systems Archives.]

appearance. Two technical factors might disturb this illusion. These are the frame rate and the degree of motion between frames. A dance floor equipped with strobe lights illuminates these points:

At low-strobe rates (e.g., 1 fps), the brightness of the empty dance floor flickers. The perception of flicker decreases as the strobe rate increases. The frequency at which flicker becomes imperceptible (the critical flicker frequency) increases with brightness. In daylight, it exceeds 60 flashes per second. This is why the refresh rate of bright computer monitors is designed to be in the 70-Hz range.

At low-strobe rates, dancers' motions appear to be discontinuous because the observer can't see what is happening between the flashes. The discontinuities become smaller as the strobe frequency increases.

Let us go back in time to the early days of motion pictures. The name "flicks" comes from this era because the films could only be projected at rates below the critical flicker frequency. In addition, actors appeared to have jerky motions in these films.

"Charlie Chaplin" has become a descriptor of low-frame rate fluoroscopy. This happens when jerky motion is seen due to appreciable motion between frames.

Neither of these effects appears in modern commercial motion pictures. Films are recorded at 24 fps. This is fast enough to produce the visual appearance of continuous motion. However, 24 fps does not exceed the critical flicker frequency. The film projector doubles the "strobe" frequency by flashing each frame twice. Visually discontinuous motion reappears if lower recording rates and high-strobe rates are used.

The relationships between object motion, recording rate, and display rate are also of significance in medical imaging. These relationships will be discussed in this and other chapters.

FILM CHANGERS

Key images have always been recorded for later review and analysis. The first recordings were made by interposing a cassette containing film and intensifying screens between the patient and the fluoroscopic screen. This practice may still be seen (with the image intensifier playing the role of the screen) in some gastrointestinal fluoroscopic systems.

It is good practice to use enough radiation to produce high-quality recordings.

Angiography requires recording at frame rates fast enough to follow the flow of contrast in the patient. Typical framing rates range from one image every few seconds up to around 10 fps. Cinefluorography (a form of motion picture technology) has been used for documenting faster processes since the dawn of the image intensifier age.

The first angiographic image receptors were cassette changers. They mechanically moved radiographic cassettes under the patient at rates up to about 2 fps. These devices were initially replaced by roll film cameras and eventually by cut film changers. The design problems included stopping the film long enough to have time for radiography and maintaining good film screen contact. These mechanical devices were large and complex. In most cases, they were mounted away from the image intensifier. This meant that the angiographer could not see the images during filming.

Film changers offered better spatial and contrast resolution than early image intensifiers. They also provided better anatomic coverage. Improvements in the size and performance of the image intensifier first lead to the replacement of film changers by film fluorographic cameras and then to digital fluorography.

CINEFLUOROGRAPHIC FILM CAMERAS

The 35-mm motion picture film format is a world standard. Film, for all its limitations, is the only image transfer medium readable anywhere in the world.

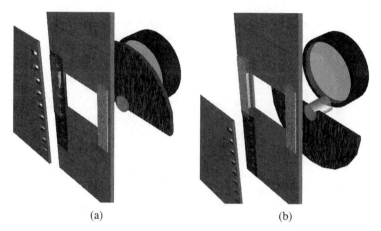

(a)   (b)

FIG. 6-2. **Schematic of internal parts of the cine-film camera.** a: The film is stationary when the shutter is opened. The X-ray beam is pulsed to form an image during this time. b: The film moves when the shutter is closed. No X rays are produced during this time.

Each image on the film is 18 mm high and 24 mm wide. This three-to-four film aspect ratio is also part of the broadcast video standard.

To avoid blur, cine film must be at rest whenever an image is recorded. The shutter interrupts the light beam when the film is advanced (Figs. 6-2 and 6-3). All motion picture cameras and projectors use intermittent motion. The loss of light (when the shutter is closed) is unimportant in a projector or in a normal motion picture camera. In a fluoroscope, irradiating the patient produces light. X rays were produced continuously in the first cine systems. This wasted half of the radiation. Pulsing the beam synchronously with the shutter's open time eliminates this waste. Patient motion blur can be reduced if the pulse time is reduced to a fraction of the shutter's open time.

The three-to-four aspect ratio of the cine-film frame is a poor match to the circular image produced by the image intensifier (Fig. 6-3). "Underframing" is one extreme example of this mismatch (Fig. 6-3A).

Underframing occurs when a short focal length camera lens is used to image the entire circle within the film frame. Early on, the inefficient use of film area caused problems with projected image brightness, granularity, and resolution. These problems have been solved over time.

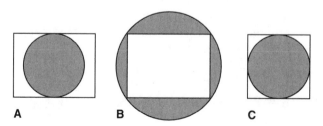

A   B   C

FIG. 6-3. **Film framing.** A: Underframed. B: Overframed. C: Medical video with a 1:1 aspect ratio.

"Overframing" is the other extreme (Fig. 6-3B). A long focal length camera lens magnifies the image such that the entire film frame is filled. Only part of the input phosphor can be seen using this setup. For radiation safety reasons, the X-ray collimators in overframed systems are set to match the irradiated and visualized fields.

Various intermediate framing protocols are also possible. These have different degrees of balance between unused film area and unused image intensifier area. One of the advantages of digital video is the ability to work with one-to-one aspect ratio images (Fig. 6-3C). This allows full visualization of the input phosphor with minimum unused video field of view.

FILM PROPERTIES

Film seldom limits the spatial resolution capabilities of fluorographic systems. The intrinsic spatial resolution of motion picture film exceeds 100 line pairs per millimeter (lp/mm). In an underframed system, a 250-mm (10-in.) field of view (FOV) input screen is reproduced on a 35-mm film frame as an 18-mm circle. The image is minified by a factor of 14. The limiting spatial resolution of good image intensifier is less than 5 lp/mm. To reproduce this resolution on film, the film stock needs to have a minimum resolution of 70 lp/mm. Proportionally, higher film resolution is required for larger FOVs.

Sensitometric Curve

Sensitometric curves describe contrast transfer properties of film. A sample curve is shown in Figure 6-4. This curve is a plot of optical density against the logarithm of the exposing light intensity. The image is a light gray in the toe region of the curve. This density is due to the film base and randomly developed film grains (fog). In this region, there is not enough light energy to form a perceptible image. The image is formed when light exposures correspond to the linear portion of the curve. The image is black in the shoulder region of the curve. All of the silver grains in the emulsion have been developed.

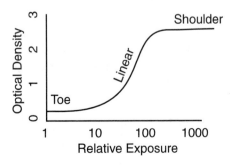

FIG. 6-4. Sensitometric curve.

Optical Density

Optical density is a meaningful imaging metric because the eye responds logarithmically to changes in light intensity. A source producing 10 times as much light than another subjectively appears to be twice as bright. Optical density (OD) is defined as

$$OD = \log_{10}(I_o/I)$$

where I_o is the intensity of the light source used to read the film and I is the intensity of the light as seen through the film.

The fraction of light transmitted through films of different optical densities is shown in Table 6-1. Inspection of this table reveals that the net optical density of two stacked pieces of film is equal to the sum of the densities of each film.

Photographic Contrast and Speed

Contrast is the difference in brightness between an object and its surroundings. An artery can only be seen if it differs from its background. The contrast of an artery as seen on film is determined by factors such as the type of "contrast medium" injected into the artery, the X-ray spectrum, and the sensitometric properties of the film.

Figure 6-5 sketches two films with different photographic contrast. The slope of the linear portion of the sensitometric curve describes film contrast. A higher contrast film (dotted line) has a steeper slope than a lower contrast film (solid line). A smaller difference in light intensity drives the higher contrast film from white to black.

Film is manufactured with different degrees of light sensitivity. A "fast" film requires less light exposure than a "slow" film. Faster films usually produce grainier images than slower films. Part of this visual effect is due to the physical structure of the film. However, the quantum nature of radiation is the major contributor to visual granularity. Image intensifiers in good condition already produce a surplus of light. Selecting a very fast film for cinefluorography will not save radiation and may actually increase image noise.

TABLE 6-1. Relation between optical density and the fraction of light transmitted through a film

	0.0	0.3	0.6	0.9
0	1.000	0.500	0.250	0.125
1	0.100	0.050	0.025	0.013
2	0.010	0.005	0.003	0.0013

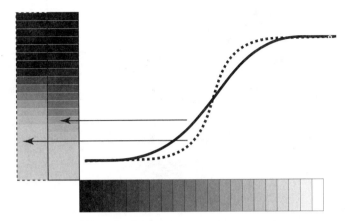

FIG. 6-5. Film Contrast. The sensitometric curves of two films are shown. The film (dotted) with the steeper slope in the linear region produces an image with more contrast. Note that brighter input steps produce more film blackening.

VIDEO SYSTEMS

In many systems, video technology provides the only access to the image intensifier's output. The same imaging chain is used for fluoroscopy, single-frame or serial fluorography, and cinefluorography. This single video channel is the technological basis for the transition from film to "filmless." The appropriate balance between patient dose and image quality is obtained by adjusting X-ray imaging properties and the system's optical diaphragm.

We are also at the cusp of the change from vacuum tube video cameras to charge-coupled device (CCD) video pickups. The corresponding transition from cathode ray tube (CRT) to flat digital displays will happen in a few years. Mass-market video users drive this change. For economic reasons, broadcast and consumer products have always been the technical bases for medical video.

Independent video pickups will disappear when the image intensifier is replaced by a direct X-ray detector.

Video Cameras

Figure 6-6 illustrates the parts of a vacuum tube video camera. Most of the cameras currently in use are based on the generic vidicon design shown in the figure.

A pattern of electrical charge is stored on the target when it is illuminated. Systematically scanning an electron beam across the target reads the charge image. Electromagnetic coils scan and focus the electron beam. Synchronization and timing are based on the frequency of the power line. Each point on the target face is interrogated at a fixed time after the synchronization pulse.

The vidicon's output is an electrical signal proportional to the light intensity at the scanned point. Figure 6-7 indicates the output voltage levels along two scan lines. The charge storage and readout processes are not perfect: The charge pattern produced by the image leaks away over time if it is not

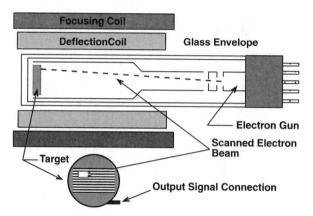

FIG. 6-6. Vidicon. Light striking the target is converted into an electrical charge distribution. Focusing and scanning coils control a scanning electron beam. The charge distribution representing the image is dissipated by the reading process.

read. The scanned readout beam leaves some residual charge in place. Fluctuations in the intensity of the scanning beam and in the readout process inject camera noise into the image.

Image storage on the target of the camera is desirable. This property permits pulsed image formation. A short pulse of radiation generates the image

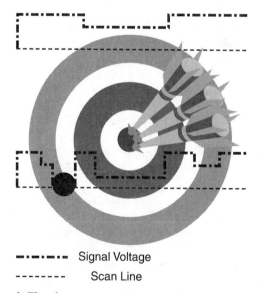

FIG. 6-7. Video signal. The charge pattern is converted into a time-varying voltage by the scanning beam. The video voltages *corresponding to two lines across the image* are shown in the figure.

in the image intensifier. The resulting charge image is stored on the target until it is read. Short pulses reduce motion unsharpness.

Residual charge has both negative and positive aspects. The next image is formed on top of a remaining portion of the previous image. This will form a blurred tail behind an object. This is called "lag." A less bright ghost artery may appear if pulsed fluoroscopy is used, and rapid motion is perpendicular to the video scan line and the axis of the artery. The right coronary artery during systole can fulfill these conditions. On the positive side, the sum of the residual and new images is less noisy than the new image itself. Low-lag cameras produce sharper images at the cost of increased image noise.

Charge-coupled device (CCD) cameras have no lag. For this reason, the noise properties of their images differ from vidicon tubes. CCD-based imaging systems usually add the equivalent of lag back into the image in the digital image processor. The visual effect is not quite the same. (Audiophiles also claim an aesthetic difference when comparing vacuum-tube and solid-state audio amplifiers.)

Camera noise has no positive aspects. Designers select cameras and other imaging components with image noise contributions that are small compared with the X-ray quantum noise. Fulfilling this requirement is the only way to ensure imaging with minimum patient dose.

Interlaced Scanning

The NTSC broadcast video standard in the United States specifies a 30-fps imaging rate. Each frame is formed of two interlaced fields, each with half the total number of scan lines. The phosphor in the display tube has a controlled amount of persistence. (A point on the phosphor continues to glow for a while after it is illuminated by the display's scanned electron beam.) This reduces flicker on home television receivers.

Figure 6-8 schematically illustrates the interlaced scanning pattern. It starts in the upper left corner of the image. A horizontal line is traced across the image. When the beam reaches the right side of the line, it is "blanked" (turned off) and deflected back to the left and down far enough to skip a line (retraced). The process is repeated until the last line in the first field is scanned. The beam is blanked and retraced to the upper left where it starts its scan in the skipped space between the two already scanned lines. The process continues until all the lines in the second field are scanned. This completes the frame. The process begins again by blanking the beam and retracing it back to the upper left corner.

The images of points in adjacent lines tend to add in the eye. The 1/60th of a second needed to return the beam to the vicinity of a given point yields an effective flicker frequency of 60 Hz. This is high enough to minimize visual image flicker. The matching persistence phosphor minimizes motion blur.

The NTSC standard is 525 horizontal lines per frame. The various retraces require some time. The result is images with 480 active scan lines. The four-to-three television aspect ratio is why the VGA computer standard specifies an output image matrix of 640×480 pixels.

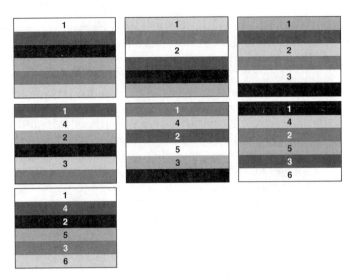

FIG. 6-8. **Interlaced scanning sequence.** The top line in the frame is scanned. One line width is skipped, and a second line is scanned. The alternating pattern is repeated until the last line in the field is scanned. Scanning the second field fills the gaps between the lines in the first field. This provides a higher flicker-frequency and permits a low-persistence phosphor for motion sharpness.

Progressive Scanning

Figure 6-9 schematically illustrates the progressive scanning pattern. Here again, the process starts in the upper left corner. When the first line is complete, the beam is retraced to the start of the next lower line (no skip). The process continues until the last line is scanned. Retracing the beam to the upper left starts the next frame.

The persistence of the phosphor cannot be increased without blurring moving objects. Perceptible image flicker will occur if a 30-fps rate (corresponding to NTSC) is used.

Progressive scanning video frame rates exceeding 70 fps eliminate perceptible flicker. Progressive scanning of the video camera in a digital imaging system is often coupled with pulsed fluoroscopic or videofluorographic acquisitions. The video beam is blanked during a single-pulse image acquisition. The charge pattern on the camera target is then read in a single pass. This process makes better use of the stored charge than does pulsed fluoroscopy followed by an interlaced readout. This process yields a modest savings in patient dose.

Experienced angiographers realize that fluoroscopy and cinefluorography are usually done at rates less than or equal to 30 fps. Flicker is reduced by digitally replaying each image several times at a high-frame rate. The process is the analog of the process previously described for motion picture projectors. The lowest usable acquisition frame rate depends on the velocity of moving objects in the scene and the observer's tolerance to jerky motion.

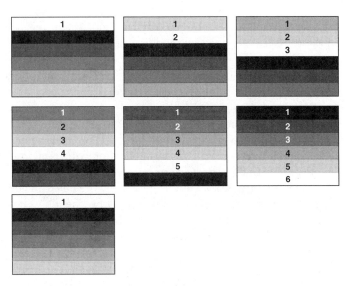

FIG. 6-9. Progressive scanning sequence. The frame is composed of one set of adjacent lines. These lines are scanned in sequence without any gaps. A high frame rate provides the necessary flicker-frequency.

Monitors

The cathode ray tube (CRT) is the standard video-viewing device. Figure 6-10 sketches the essential elements of its construction. An electron beam is generated by an electron gun containing the tube's cathode (cathode rays). This beam is scanned across a phosphor screen located inside the faceplate.

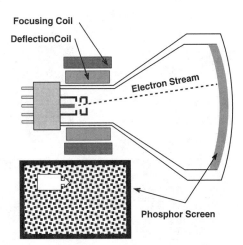

FIG. 6-10. Cathode ray tube (CRT). A focused electron beam is scanned across the face of the tube by the coils. The intensity of the beam is modulated by the video signal voltage. The electron beam causes a phosphor to fluoresce. The varying beam intensity "paints" an image on the phosphor.

These electrons cause the phosphor to fluoresce at the point of contact. Local brightness is controlled by modulating the intensity of the electron beam.

A color CRT uses groups of red, green, and blue phosphors. Three separate electron guns are used to drive their respective color phosphors. Adjusting the intensity of each primary color generates a range of colors. In a color CRT, combining red, green, and blue signals generates gray-scale images.

A monochrome CRT uses a single phosphor. The designer selects the phosphor that produces the appropriate color of fluorescent light and possesses the appropriate lag. A long-lag phosphor will exhibit less flicker and more motion blur than a short-lag phosphor.

The brightness of a CRT is limited by the electron gun's ability to generate a high-power finely focused beam and by the phosphor's ability to handle electron beam heating without degradation. Phosphors degrade with time and use. Monitor brightness should be checked as part of the quality assurance program.

CRT brightness is much less than that of a radiographic–view box or a cine projector. As previously noted, the spatial and contrast sensitivity of the eye varies with light level. Different image processing algorithms are needed to match hard- and soft-copy images of the same scene.

The electron beam in the CRT is scanned synchronously with the beam in the video camera (Fig. 6-11). When broadcast standards were initially established, sync-lock between a broadcast studio camera and many widely dispersed home receivers was a significant technical achievement. This is why timing and frame rates are based on the very stable frequency of the AC supplied by the power company.

CRTs are being replaced by solid-state displays. The technology that is deployed for a particular application is selected after the amount of motion

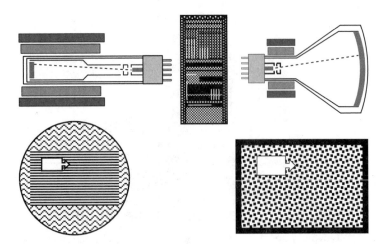

FIG. 6-11. Synchronized scanning. The position of the writing beam in the CRT is synchronized in time and position with the reading beam in the camera tube. The stable power line frequency maintains synchronization between a studio camera and home receivers.

expected in the scene, image size, and cost is considered. At the time of this writing, solid-state displays did not quite have the gray-scale display capability appropriate for medical diagnosis.

Scan Converters

It may be necessary to convert a video signal from one format to another. This might be done to bring a European sports event to a United States television network. A specialized device, not surprisingly called a scan converter, is used for this purpose. The scan converter has proven to be a useful medical imaging device.

The original scan converter was a vacuum tube similar to a CRT. An input electron beam writes the input image as a charge pattern on a storage mesh. An independent readout electron beam simultaneously reads the charge distribution in a manner similar to that of a vidicon. Scan conversion is accomplished because there is no need to drive the input and output sides of the device with the same video format. As indicated in Figure 6-12, the scan converter can generate output images that differ in both lines per frame and frame rate from the input images.

The modern scan converter is a digital image memory. The image is written into the memory using the input video format, and readout of the memory is accomplished using the output video format. The stored digital image is nonvolatile. This gives the added flexibility of generating multiple output frames for each input frame. This enables fluoroscopy and digital cinefluorography at low-acquisition–frame rates with simultaneous display at frame rates high enough to eliminate image flicker. The end of this sequence is last-image hold. The last fluoroscopic image stays in the scan converter's memory and is continuously replayed until a new fluoroscopic session is initiated.

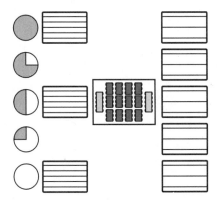

FIG. 6-12. Scan converter. Images are written into the device using the input frame format and frame rate. Images emerging from the device can be in another format and rate. One major use of a scan converter is conversion of high-resolution medical images into broadcast format.

MINI COURSE

Cameras and displays need to be matched to both the dynamics of the medical situation and the physiology of the observers' eye.

The video chain (with digital processing) is currently the only image channel used for both fluoroscopy and fluorography.

Technical details of United States and European medical imaging chains differ because of different broadcast standards.

SECTION THREE

Digital Images

7

Digital Images*

*Based on an article originally appearing in Balter, S., Fundamentals of Digital Images, *RadioGraphics* 1993 13:129–141. Used with permission of the Radiological Society of North America.

ANALOG-TO-DIGITAL CONVERSION

Analog images, such as visual scenes and photographs, are continuous in both position and brightness (see Fig. 7-1). A digital image is divided into a set of spatial domains called pixels. Each pixel is filled with the same uniform brightness. The brightness level in each pixel is chosen from a discrete set.

The eye itself is an analog-to-digital converter. The mosaic of image receptors in the retina determines pixel size. Each receptor encodes light level as a series of neurological pulses. The retina and its supporting neural network are digital image processing tools.

Figure 7-2 illustrates basic concepts. In the first step of the digitization process, this analog scene is divided into 16 pixels. The average brightness in each pixel is measured. This value is used to fill the area covered by that pixel.

The spatial digitization process begins with the input device. For example, a video image is composed of a number of lines. The width of a line sets the pixel height. The distance over which the video signal is averaged along a line determines the pixel width.

The number and arrangement of the pixels in an image is fixed by the imaging hardware. Each individual pixel is usually a square. Images with a four-to-three aspect ratio (e.g., conventional television, 35-mm slides) have a corresponding four-to-three ratio of pixel columns to rows. Fluoroscopic images have a one-to-one aspect ratio. The corresponding digital matrix is a square.

The effective size of a pixel increases with an increasing field–of–view (FOV) and decreases with a increasing number of pixels in the digital matrix. Table 7-1 shows examples of this relationship.

The brightness used to fill a pixel is chosen from a list of discreet values. In the digital domain, it is convenient to use lists that have sizes based on the binary number system (Table 7-2).

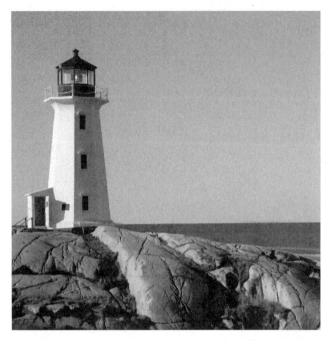

FIG. 7-1. Original "analog" image. This image was originally captured on color photographic film. It was necessary to digitize the negative for reproduction in this book. [Peggy's Cove, Nova Scotia, Canada. Photograph taken by author.]

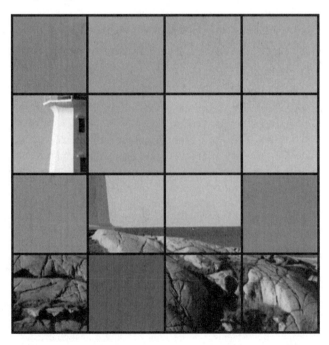

FIG. 7-2. Conversion of an analog to a digital image. Th e "analog" image has been divided into 16 pixels. The average brightness in each portion of the original scene is represented by a uniform gray level filling the corresponding pixel.

TABLE 7-1. Relationships between matrix size, pixel size, and field–of–view

| | Field–of–view at the image receptor | | |
| | 25 cm | 18 cm | 13 cm |
Matrix size	Pixel size (mm)		
128 × 128	1.95	1.41	1.02
256 × 256	0.98	0.70	0.51
512 × 512	0.49	0.35	0.25
1024 × 1024	0.24	0.18	0.13

TABLE 7-2. Available shades of gray as a function of number of bits per pixel

Bits per pixel	Shades of Gray	Bits per pixel	Shades of Gray
1	2	7	128
2	4	8	256
3	8	9	1,024
4	16	10	2,048
5	32	11	4,096
6	64	12	8,192

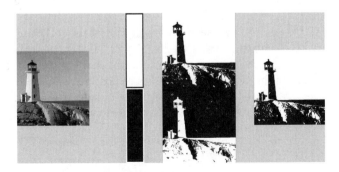

FIG. 7-3. One-bit analog-to-digital converter. The brightness in each pixel of the original image is compared with a reference 50% level. Pixels exceeding this level are stored as binary level (1). These pixels appear bright in the upper center image. These pixels are printed as white in the final image (on the *right*). Pixels below this level are stored as binary level (0). These pixels appear bright in the lower center image. They are printed as black in the final image.

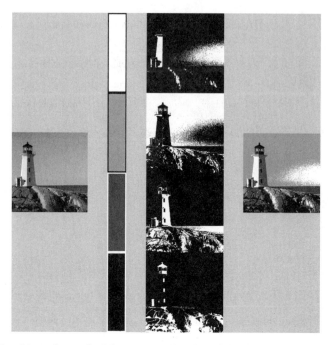

FIG. 7-4. Two-bit analog-to-digital converter. Pixels with brightness below 25% are stored as binary level (00). These pixels appear bright in the lowest center image. They are printed as black in the final image. Pixels with brightness between 25% and 50% are stored as binary level (01). They are printed as dark gray. Pixels with brightness between 50% and 75% are stored as binary level (10). These are printed as light gray. Pixels with brightness exceeding 75% are stored as binary level (11). They are printed as white.

The pixels in a one-bit image are either black or white. Figure 7-3 illustrates the one-bit conversion process. The brightness in each pixel is measured by the analog-to-digital converter (ADC). Pixels exceeding 50% of the maximum brightness of the scene are encoded as white. Pixels with less brightness are encoded as black.

Figure 7-4 illustrates a two-bit gray-scale encoding process. Brightness is encoded into four steps 0–25, 26–50, 51–75, and 76–100% of maximum. These steps are represented by black, dark gray, light gray, or white. Each additional bit doubles the number of possible levels. An eight-bit process provides 256 levels. These levels are close enough to each other for the digitization steps to be imperceptible to the human eye.

Moore's law of computing: The cost of key computer resources drops by a factor of two every 18 months.

MATRIX SIZE

Figure 7-5 illustrates the influence of matrix size on image quality. The pixel matrix sizes are 1024 × 1024, 256 × 256, and 64 × 64. Small pixels at normal

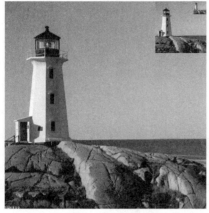
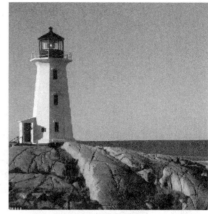

(a) 1024 x 1024 (8 bit)   (b) 256 x 256 (8 bit)

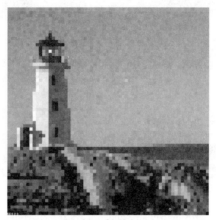

(c) 64 x 64 (8 bit)

FIG. 7-5. Matrix size. The original scene is digitized using pixel matrices of 1024 × 1024 (a), 256 × 256 (b), and 64 × 64 (c). The brightness is digitized to 256 levels. The inserts in the upper left corner of (a) represent the relative computer resources needed to manage the 256 and 64 pixel matrices.

viewing distances are individually below the resolution limit of the eye. Physiological averaging produces a visually continuous image.

The load on the technological infrastructure (e.g., storage space and transmission time) increases with the number of pixels in an image. The 1024 × 1024 matrix requires 16 times as many resources than the 256 × 256 image. The 64 × 64 matrix requires 1/16 as many resources. The inset in Figure 7-5a illustrates this point.

Sharpness of the original analog image determines the maximum useful matrix size (Fig. 7-6). There is a blur radius associated with image unsharpness.

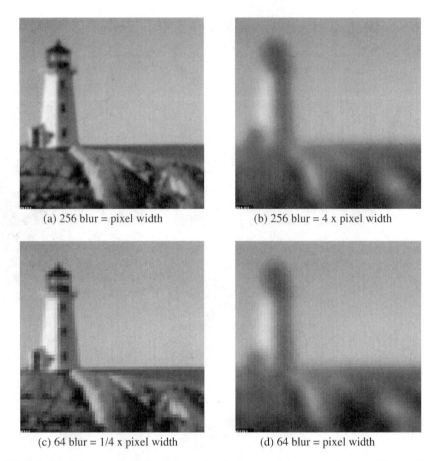

(a) 256 blur = pixel width   (b) 256 blur = 4 x pixel width

(c) 64 blur = 1/4 x pixel width   (d) 64 blur = pixel width

FIG. 7-6. Useful matrix size depends on the sharpness of the original image. The smallest useful pixel size (largest matrix) is comparable to the blur in the underlying image. The image is digitized to a 256 matrix in a and b and to a 64 matrix in c and d. The blur radius in a and c is comparable to the pixel width in a. The blur radius in b and d is comparable to the pixel width in c.

If the blur radius is small compared with the pixel size, then the digital image sharpness is limited by the pixels. If there is a large degree of blur, then the sharpness is limited by the original image.

Magnifying an image before digitization (e.g., using the image intensifier's zoom mode) decreases the effective pixel size because the same number of pixels covers a smaller anatomic area. Magnifying each pixel in an image after digitization covers the smaller anatomic area with fewer primary pixels. The effect of either zoom mode on sharpness remains dependent on the relation between primary pixel size and blur in the original image.

BIT DEPTH

Figure 7-7 illustrates the effect of bit depth on image quality. Decreasing the number of discreet brightness levels decreases the technical resources needed for image handling and display. Artificial contours appear when the difference in brightness between adjacent levels is large enough to be perceptible. This is seen in the sky region of Figure 7-7c.

The maximum usable bit depth is noise dependent (Fig. 7-8). If the amplitude of the noise is small relative to the digital brightness steps, then the

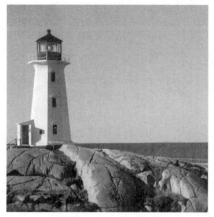
(a) 8 bit (1024 matrix)

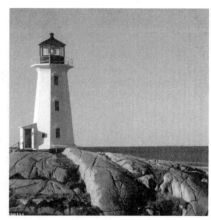
(b) 5 bit (1024 matrix)

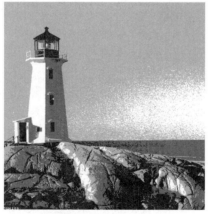
(c) 2 bit (1024 matrix)

FIG. 7-7. Effect of bit depth. This 1024 image has been digitized to 8 bits, 256 levels (a); 5 bits, 32 levels (b); and 2 bits, 4 levels (c). The brightness steps are imperceptible in a, perceptible in b, and obvious in c. The visible boundary seen in the sky in c is called a pseudocontour.

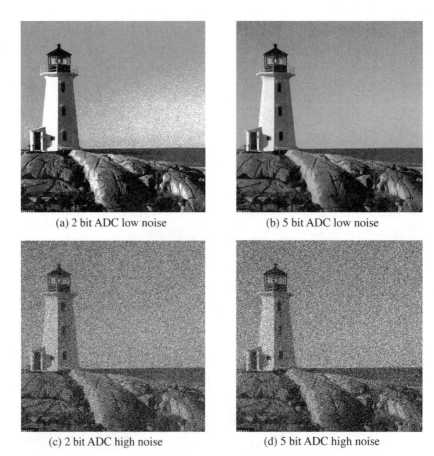

(a) 2 bit ADC low noise   (b) 5 bit ADC low noise

(c) 2 bit ADC high noise   (d) 5 bit ADC high noise

FIG. 7-8. The useful bit depth depends on image noise. Before digitization, a small amount of noise has been added to the two-bit image (a) and the five bit image (b). The pseudo-contours in b remain visible under low noise conditions. The large amount of noise present before digitization in c and d masks the difference in bit depths between these two images.

number of bits in the ADC will determine the brightness variations in the image. Relatively large noise amplitude will dominate the ADC and therefore control image appearance.

SINGLE PIXEL PROCESSING

Manipulating the brightness levels of the pixels changes the overall brightness and visual contrast of a digital image. The ADC determines the initial brightness of each pixel. These input values are transformed into output values by means of a look-up table (LUT). The LUT is the digital equivalent of film's sensometric curve. LUTs are used to correct for nonlinearity of film, monitors, and the eye. They are also used to alter image aesthetics. All digital images are processed by means of a LUT. The acceptability and perhaps the utility of an image are strongly dominated by the LUT.

The difference between clinical LUTs can be either obvious or subtle. Figure 7-9 illustrates some extreme LUTs. These have been chosen to demonstrate the effect of LUT on imaging in a manner that is independent of the printing process. A linear LUT was used to prepare the image in Figure 7-9A. This LUT does not affect the appearance of the image. Figure 7-9D demonstrates the effect of an inverse LUT. Objects, such as the windows, that are black in the original scene are transformed to white. The left-hand side of the tower is transformed from white to black. Light-gray objects become dark gray and vice versa.

Figure 7-9B and Figure 7-9C illustrate some LUTs that can be produced digitally. In B, blackish and whitish objects are reproduced at increased contrast. Tones in the original scene ranging from light to dark gray are reproduced as a monotone (e.g., sky and rock shading). No contrast remains in this portion of the image. In C, blackish and whitish objects have been reproduced with a further increase in contrast. However, the midscale objects have been inverted. Note that windows remain black and that the sea is now brighter than the sky.

A "natural" looking digital image has undergone at least as much image processing as an "enhanced image."

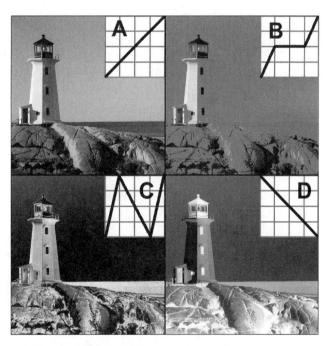

FIG. 7-9. Effect of look-up table (LUT). A: The input and output images are identical. B: Contrast has been increased for originally low (0–25%) and high (76–100%) pixels. Original (26–75%) pixels are reproduced at a uniform brightness. There is no contrast in this region. C: Contrast has been further increased in the 0–25% and 76–100% regions. Contrast is reversed in the intermediate region. Note the contrast reversal between the sea and sky. D: Inverse linear transformation. Note that the windows are now white.

SINGLE-IMAGE PROCESSING

The numerical value of the contents of a pixel can be replaced with a controlled combination of the values found in the original pixel and in other pixels in the image. Some of the multi-pixel operations commonly found in medical imaging are blur, sharpening, and zoom.

Blur

Digital images are blurred to mask cosmetic defects and noise. Blur reduces image sharpness. Each pixel value is sequentially replaced by an average of the value in that pixel and its neighbors. The number of pixels included in the average governs the degree of blur. Adjusting the weighting factors of pixels at different distances controls the nature of the blur. The blur shown in Figure 7-5 was produced by this means.

Digital Zoom

An image can be magnified either by the use of the same number of output pixels or by increasing the number of the same-size pixels used to display the image. Image magnification cannot improve the sharpness of the original image. However, magnification can improve the perceived sharpness of small objects by bringing them to the region of peak spatial sensitivity of the eye. The same effect can be obtained by changing viewing distance. Image minification improves the perceptibility of large diffuse objects. This effect is well known to radiologists looking for lung nodules.

A physically larger monitor fills the display with a fixed number of pixels. The television display in the scoreboard of a ball field has no more pixels than the pocket receiver carried by a fan sitting in the stands.

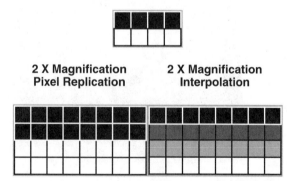

FIG. 7-10. **Digital magnification.** An image is digitally magnified by filling several pixels in the output image with the contents of one pixel in the input image. In *Pixel Replication*, all of the corresponding new pixels are filled with the same brightness. In *Interpolation*, an average value of the original pixel and its surroundings is used to fill the intermediate new pixels. This figure illustrates linear interpolation.

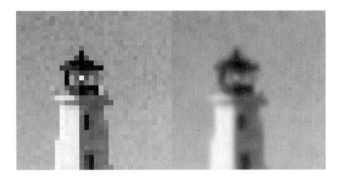

FIG. 7-11. Figure 7–11. **Appearance of different magnification methods.** Pixel replication produces a blocky image appearance. Interpolation produces a blurred image. The visibility of interpolation blur is affected by the amount of blur in the original image.

A physically larger device can also be filled with more pixels. Using several display pixels to represent each pixel in the original image magnifies an image. There are two ways to do this: pixel replication and interpolation (Figs. 7-10 and 7-11) Pixel replication fills each of the several pixels in the magnified image with the value of the single original pixel. This can result in a blocky looking image. Interpolation fills those pixels in the magnified matrix corresponding to the pixels in the original matrix with the original values. The additional pixels are filled using values interpolated between the original values. This process provides a smooth transition between pixels. It may also increase image blur.

Sharpening (Unsharp Mask Process)

The visual sharpness of an image can be modified by first forming a blurred version (unsharp mask) of the original image and then subtracting the mask from the original image. The appearance of the resulting image is determined by the blur radius used to form the mask and the relative intensities of the original and masked images that are combined to form the resultant image (Fig. 7-12).

MULTIPLE IMAGE PROCESSING

One can also combine two or more digital images. Subtracting one image from another reveals the difference between the two images. Adding images to one another reduces noise.

Image Subtraction

Detecting the difference between two images can be useful. The overall process is illustrated in Figure 7-13. The two images (A and B) differ by the absence of the guardrail and the searchlight. (It is left to the readers imagination as to

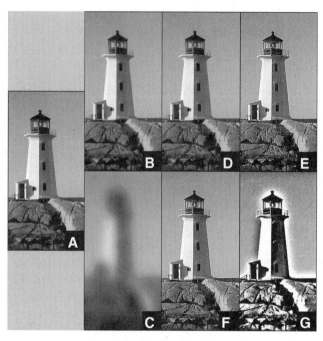

FIG. 7-12. Unsharp masking. A blurred copy of the original scene (A) is generated by optical or digital means. This is called a *mask*. Subtracting the mask from the original image generates the final image. Different degrees of blur (B and C) and different weighting of the original and mask image produce the four images shown in (D–F). The same weighting factor is used for D and F and E and G.

how image A was produced.) Each of these images contains an amount and distribution of noise equivalent to the X-ray quantum noise content of a typical radiograph.

The subtraction process removes objects that are identical in both images. Pixels with no difference are usually set to a medium brightness as part of the subtraction process. Depending on its appearance in the original images and on the subtraction order, a difference appears that is either lighter or darker than the reference value. This is best seen in Figure 7-13E.

Subtraction is performed to reveal subtle differences between the images. The visibility of these differences is improved by increasing the contrast of the subtraction image. Figure 7-13C is an image of the raw subtraction. D–F have had the same degree of contrast increase.

Figure 7-13E illustrates the effect of subtracting two noise-free images. The random nature of noise means that the noise pattern is not identical in the two images. X-ray noise does not subtract. The effect of this is shown before and after contrast expansion in Figures 7-13C and 7-13D.

The subtraction process does not work if the images contain too much quantum noise (Fig. 7-13F) This is caused by imaging with insufficient image receptor dose. Subtraction in images having subtle differences requires more dose per frame than that needed for viewing gross differences or unsubtracted images.

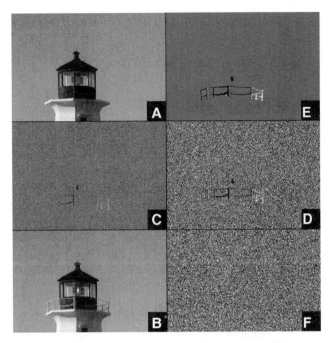

FIG. 7-13. Subtraction reveals differences. The differences are the lack of a safety rail and the absence of the searchlight in A compared with B. The raw difference image is shown in C. Visibility of the difference is improved by increasing image contrast. The noise contents of images A and B are added in the subtracted image. Increasing image contrast also increases the visibility of noise. E illustrates a noise-free subtraction. The selected subtraction order converted white objects only appearing in B as black and visa versa. D illustrates C with the same degree of contrast stretch as in E. F illustrates a high noise image with contrast stretch. The subtle subtraction signals are masked by the noise.

Subtraction is usually used to reveal image changes over time (temporal subtraction). Other forms of subtraction are technically possible and may be of clinical interest. For example, an energy difference image is formed by subtracting two images formed with different portions of the X-ray spectrum. Appropriate selection of the weighting factors emphasizes or suppresses the presence of calcium.

Images used for subtraction require more dose per frame than those viewed without subtraction.

Image Addition

X-ray images are dominated by X-ray quantum noise. Adding images together effectively combines the radiation flux in the separate images (Fig. 7-14). This reduces image noise.

This process is very acceptable for imaging a static scene. However, a moving object occupies a different position in each image. Now, when the images are added, the resultant has multiple images of the moving object (Fig. 7-15).

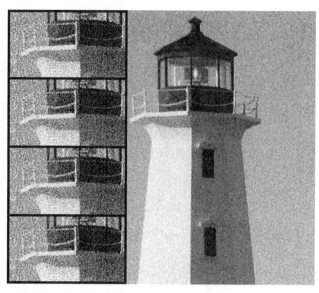

FIG. 7-14. Image addition reduces noise. Four images of the same scene are added to each other. The lighthouse pixels combine in all images. The noise fluctuations average to a lower visual noise level. Four images of the same X-ray quantum-limited scene combine to reduce the noise appearance by a factor of two.

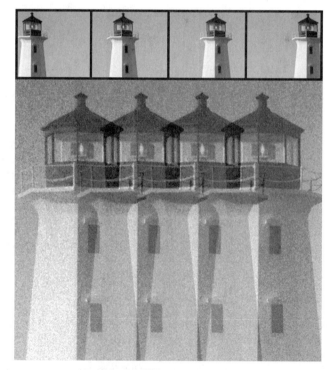

FIG. 7-15. Image addition blurs a moving object. A moving object does not sum together when images are added. The multiple exposure appearance of this scene is due to the large displacement of the tower between images. A small displacement produces a blurred image. Note that visual noise is reduced.

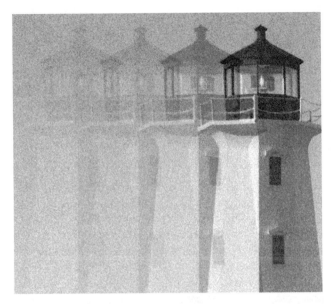

FIG. 7-16. **Recursive filtering (80%) can reduce noise.** Note the multiple exposure effect. A fraction of the previous image is added to the new image. The oldest part of the image fades out as this recursive process is repeated. The recursion percentage is 80% in this example.

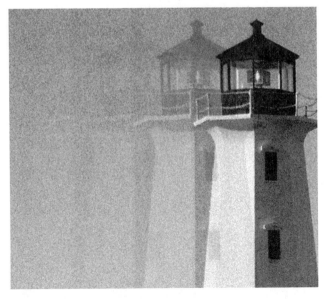

FIG. 7-17. **Recursive filtering (50%).** In this example, the recursion percentage is 50%. The older part of the image fades more rapidly than in Figure 7-16. However, there is also less noise integration in this scene.

Recursive filtering is a form of image addition. The trail of multiple copies of the moving object is reduced by adding a fraction of the previous image to the new image (Figs. 7-16 and 7-17). Adding a large recursive fraction increases the effective number of frames in the average. This provides a large degree of noise reduction at the cost of significant motion blur. The appropriate degree of recursive filtering represents a balance between noise and blur.

CLINICAL IMAGE PROCESSING SETS

This brief chapter can only serve to introduce the rich and growing world of digital imaging tools. Appropriate processing improves the perceptibility of clinically important information. Image processing sets tuned to answer specific clinical questions are increasingly available. However, image processing optimized to answer one question may mask the presence of an equally important but unsuspected condition. There is seldom time enough to use multiple processing sets on each image of every patient. The selection of appropriate image processing sets is ultimately one of the many arts inherent in the practice of medicine.

Digital fluoro systems are delivered with a "factory" image processing set. Many other sets are available.

MINI COURSE

Doubling the intrinsic spatial resolution of a digital image increases its bit size by a factor of four. The maximum useful resolution is usually determined by conventional imaging factors.

The number of bits needed to describe a pixel depends on the acceptable noise level in the image. Hence, more bits per pixel are needed in images used for subtraction.

The visual appearance of the image is determined by the look-up table and other image processing factors.

8

Image Networks

INTRODUCTION

The management of radiographic images has moved from traditional files of films into the digital domain of electronic archives and video displays. One of the important benefits is the ability to maintain the file of master images in an inviolate archive. Exact digital copies of these images are generated when required for viewing or transfer.

A useful imaging network needs to only perform a few basic functions. These are image input, image demographic input, image storage, database management, and image output. Such networks have been given the generic name "picture archiving and communication systems" (PACS). Systems that are designed to handle cardiac cine must meet technical requirements that are much different from those needed to manage a hospital's file of chest radiographs. In this chapter, the designation R-PACS refers to general-purpose radiological systems.

This chapter introduces the organization and workflow found in PACS suitable for angiography and cardiology. A system suitable for both is denoted as CV-PACS. V-PACS and C-PACS denote systems specialized for noncardiac and cardiac interventional systems, respectively.

Every interventional lab has some form of CV-PACS. These range from conventional film-based systems to elaborate electronic networks. Proper implementation of CV-PACS should improve the efficiency of a well-organized laboratory. Technology is unlikely to bring order out of chaos.

IMAGE FORMATS AND STANDARDS

Formats

Digital images come in a variety of formats. These are characterized by matrix size and bit depth. The required format depends on the ultimate use of the images.

Vascular images are typically 1024 × 1024 or 2048 × 2048 at either 10 or 12 bits. The large matrix size is needed to provide adequate spatial resolution across a large field of view. The 10- to 12-bit pixel depth allows sufficient contrast resolution for subtraction. A typical vascular interventional procedure will generate up to 100 images. Some neurointerventional procedures generate many hundreds of images. For planning purposes, an average vascular study requires 200 megabytes of storage before compression.

Cardiac images are typically 512 × 512 × 8 bit. This provides appropriate spatial resolution for the 25-cm and smaller cardiac image intensifiers. The eight-bit pixel depth is sufficient for viewing nonsubtracted images of contrast-filled structures. A typical cardiac procedure generates a few thousand images. For planning purposes, an average cardiac study requires 600 megabytes of storage before compression.

Larger matrix sizes and bit depths are needed for digital radiography (DR). Here, the tasks include very large fields of view and the viewing of nonsubtracted images of subtle anatomic contrast. A DR study seldom includes more than 10 images. Chest radiographs are usually half of the total case volume. This lowers the average. The planning number for DR is 10 megabytes per study. The reader is referred to standard textbooks dealing with R-PACS.

Digital Imaging and Communications in Medicine (DICOM)

Digital fluorographs are usually presented to image-handling devices encoded in *a* DICOM format. The image format inside the angiographic system's image processor is whatever meets the manufacturer's engineering requirements.

The DICOM standard prescribes a specific way of generating logical image formats. Note the italic "*a*" in the previous paragraph. DICOM provides a great deal of flexibility. Many formats fall under the DICOM umbrella. Indeed, one of the virtues of DICOM is its ability to accommodate different formats.

An imager capable of handling and displaying one DICOM format may or may not be capable of handling images in similar formats and is not expected to handle any DICOM image. (One would not always expect to be able to view a color nuclear stress scan on a viewer designed for chest radiographs.) DICOM also allows physical devices (e.g., printers, storage devices) to announce their capabilities over a network in a standard manner.

Cardiac and vascular image structures are similar enough to allow a common discussion. CV-PACS are available to handle both varieties. DICOM files are logically organized with a hierarchy of "image," "run," and "study." A DICOM file contains a header, and the images are organized into runs and studies. The header contains a technical description of the images, patient and facility information, image processing settings, and other technical parameters needed for optimum viewing. In future versions of the standard, physiological and other clinical data can also be included. File integrity and authenticity might be certified by including appropriately encrypted fields in the header.

The "physical format" of an image is a description of the physical medium on which the image is recorded. An image can be written in the same logical format onto many different physical media. Exact digital copies of the image used to produce the figures in this book have been stored in the computer's hard disk, on a floppy disk, on a recordable CD and on a magnetic tape. One may also store an image on the same physical medium in a variety of logical formats. (The images were stored in at least three different logical formats during the production process of this book.)

Conformance statements are available for physical devices and logical image formats. Examination of conformance statements will identify those entities that are capable of working together. One further complication is the presence of "private" fields in DICOM headers. Such fields give a manufacturer the possibility of transferring specific information between their own devices; for example, a particular look-up table from an angiographic room can be transferred to a freestanding viewing station. However, DICOM images are intended to be viewable without access to the private fields.

The DICOM CD-R format used in cardiology is a unique combination of physical and logical formats. It is specified as a means of mechanically transferring digital cardiac images between pieces of imaging hardware. The disk is intended to be as universally exchangeable as a roll of 35-mm cine film. This format provides great flexibility. A manufacturer may place proprietary tracks on a disk in addition to the DICOM track. Some manufacturers used highly compressed tracks to work around the slow reading speed of early CD players. The disadvantage is the loss of space on the disk for the DICOM data set. Private fields, often found in the header, may cause unexpected difficulties when there are incompatibilities between the writing and reading software. The DICOM cardiac disk has been successful in its intended purpose. The interchangeability of disks between different manufacturers' systems has increased over time because improved computer hardware lessens the designers' dependence on private fields and proprietary tracks. The extension of the CD to archival use has occurred, although this is not formally part of the DICOM specification.

NETWORKING BASICS

Conventional Workflow

It is useful to follow the workflow of conventional cine film to understand the organization of an electronic system. The flow of angiographic images is similar. Figure 8-1 illustrates a conventional film-based C-PACS.

Demographic information (e.g., patient name, hospital number, lab number, referring physician) is supplied via an examination request. In most cardiac labs, basic demographic information, written in lead, is then placed on the patient and fluorographed onto the film (see filled arrow in Fig. 8-1). This provides an unambiguous link between the patient and the images.

At the conclusion of the case, demographic information is written into the logbook of the lab, and the film is placed into a film can. The film can, labeled for visual retrieval, is placed on a "current cases" shelf. Eventually the can will be moved to a long-term storage area. This move is documented in the log of the lab.

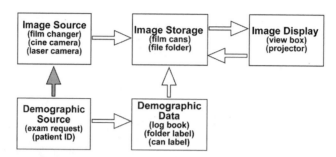

FIG. 8-1. **Image workflow using film as the information carrier.** The film might come from a film changer, cine-camera, or be hard-copy prints of digital images.

When a current case is needed, the film can is taken from the shelf and brought to the cine projector. An old case usually flows from the archive to the shelf to the projector. Various log-out systems are used to track the location of out-of-file films. The film is returned to the file after use. Before this happens, filmed demographics are used to verify that the correct film is in the correct can.

DIGITAL CV-PACS

Every imaging department has a PACS system; it might be manual, electronic, or partially each.

DICOM CD-Based C-PACS

A simple C-PACS can be organized around DICOM CDs (Fig. 8-2). Demographic data are typed into the angiographic system at the start of the study.

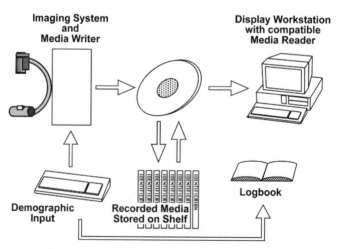

FIG. 8-2. **Image workflow.** DICOM CDs or proprietary media are used in place of conventional film.

The system writes a CD containing demographics and images at the conclusion of the study. The occasional very long study can be written on multiple disks. Human readable identifiers (e.g., patient name and lab number) are manually placed on the disk or on its caddy. The disk is then stored on a file shelf. When the patient's images are needed, the disk is removed from the file and carried to a reader. The disk is manually refilled when it is no longer needed. The database describing the disk file may include some degree of automation or might simply be the logbook of the laboratory. It should be noted that the official role of the DICOM CD is for image transfer. Archiving is currently an "off-label" use.

A CD-based V-PACS does not exist simply because there is no current DICOM specification for vascular CDs.

Networked PACS

A networked CV-PACS (Fig. 8-3) replaces much of the manual effort with communication cables, robotics that handle storage of media, and an internal database. Demographics are typed into the imaging system's computer. At the conclusion of the case, the imaging system creates a DICOM file. This file contains the DICOM header and images.

The file is transferred to an image server using the connecting network. Patient demographics are written into the server's database. The demographic information might enter via a hospital information system (HIS), the angiographic imaging system, or a CV-PACS terminal.

Images are stored in the active file. When the active file is full, old cases are transferred to an on-line archive. When the archive is full, the oldest cases

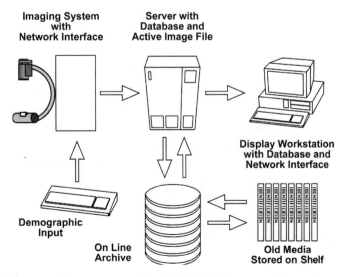

FIG. 8-3. Image workflow in a networked C-PACS. Electronic links replace most of the manual transfer steps. Older cases may be stored on a simple shelf.

are ejected and manually stored on a shelf. Technical increases in storage density will eventually eliminate the need for "shelf" storage.

Viewing a case starts with a search of the database. If necessary, the case is recalled into the active file from the archive or the shelf. A copy of the case is then transferred over the network to the display workstation. It will take more time to obtain an older case from the archive or shelf.

Ideally, master copies of the cases never leave the CV-PACS central storage area. Electronic or physical replicas (working copies) are transferred to the readers or elsewhere. The use of disposable replicas of noncirculating masters is the most important feature of digital archives such as CV-PACS. The value of protecting the masters from being lost is self-evident. Creating multiple working copies permits multiple simultaneous accesses to the clinical information.

HARDWARE

Image Acquisition

There are three main paths available for the transfer of data from the angiographic system into CV-PACS (Fig. 8-4). These are the DICOM-CD, video capture, or digital transfer. DICOM-CD transfer involves the preparation of a disk by the angiographic system and its manual insertion into a reader attached to the C-PACS internal storage. After this, the transfer disk is no longer needed for the archive.

Video capture of an available television signal provides the second path into CV-PACS. Most angiographic systems have two video signals available. The first potential connecting point is between the television camera in the image intensifier and the angiographic digital image processor. The second connecting point is between the image processor and the angiographic tele-

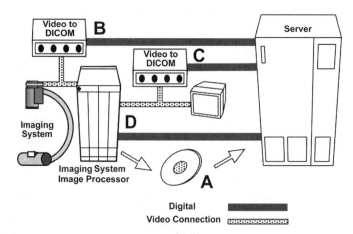

FIG. 8-4. Images can be transferred by several means. A: DICOM CD. B: Video capture from the camera looking at the image intensifier. C: Video capture from the line connecting to the in lab viewing monitor. D: Direct digital connection.

vision monitors. Tapping the signal at the image intensifier by-passes all of the image processing provided by the X-ray manufacturer. Acquiring video from the image processors' output means that data have gone through an analog-to-digital transformation and have been processed in a way that prepares the image for the angiographic monitors. In both cases, the image is redigitized by a second analog-to-digitital converter located in the CV-PACS.

Direct digital transfer of information requires that the angiographic system and CV-PACS share a mutually compatible communication channel. It also requires the CV-PACS to properly interpret the logical format supplied by the angiographic system. Newer systems offer the option of a "DICOM output" that meets these requirements. Interface computers are available for older systems. These devices accept the proprietary communications and logical formats supplied by the angiographic system and reformat the data into the expected DICOM format.

Image Servers

The client-server model is used to illustrate a common CV-PACS network structure. Other network structures are also available. These structures can also provide satisfactory clinical performance.

One or more computers provide central file management for a client-server network. These are the servers. Client workstations send information to and receive information from the server. In a CV-PACS environment, the cardiologist's viewing station, the angiographic system's DICOM interface computer, and so forth are all clients.

A small network might have a single server. Its failure will disable the network. Servers used for critical systems have their own spare components already installed. The most obvious of these is an uninterruptible power supply (UPS). The UPS can power the server for a short while with its batteries. The server's power requirements and the time needed to restore power determine the size of the UPS.

Operating software, the database, and images are stored on hard disks. Servers usually incorporate a redundant array of independent disks (RAID). A portion of each byte is stored on each of the RAID disks. When a disk fails, the server immediately reconstructs its data and writes the data onto a spare disk. Many RAIDs permit "hot swapping." A defective disk can be removed and replaced without turning the server off.

The server has space to store a limited number of cases in its RAID. This is a matter of economics. RAIDs are the fastest and most expensive forms of mass storage available in the CV-PACS. A good balance is to have a RAID big enough to store 1–2 weeks' worth of cases. Remaining "on-line" cases are stored in a less expensive secondary device. Less RAID capacity is needed when fast secondary storage is used.

A single server supports many clients. Servers need to be able to communicate fast enough to avoid slowing the work of the clients. The principal load on a CV-PACS server is image management. As the number of active clients increases, different server hardware and software architectures will have different behaviors. Servers might either uniformly slow the frame rate delivered to all the clients or supply a high-frame rate to a few clients at the expense of a very low-frame rate delivered to other clients.

Secondary Storage (Image Archives)

The image archive provides on-line storage at a lower cost per case than the RAID. Robotic handling of individual pieces of storage media is found in image archives. Mechanical handling time significantly increases the response time of the image archive relative to the RAID.

Digital tape (DT, a form of magnetic tape) and magneto-optical disks (MOD) are currently the predominant storage technologies. CDV-R, a high-density recordable compact disk, is emerging. DT is the densest (cases per square foot of archive space) and least expensive (dollars per case) of these technologies. DT may require more maintenance than other storage technologies.

Image archives are available in several sizes. The appropriate size depends on the clinical volume of the laboratory and the time pattern of patient returns. Thirteen months' worth of storage provides enough space for annual follow-ups plus a margin for scheduling delays.

Eventually, all of the media storage slots in the archive may be filled. The oldest disks or tapes can be ejected and manually stored on a shelf. The index to these cases remains in the database. A disk or tape is manually reinserted into the archive when access to its cases is required.

There is a good chance that media will never have to be removed from the archive. Evolving technology is expected to provide more responsive, denser, and less expensive storage means. The existing archive hardware can be upgraded. This can be illustrated by using MODs as an example: The present 2.5-gigabyte disks can be replaced with 5-gigabyte models. New read-write drives usually work with old disks. One can replace the drives and then insert 5-gigabyte disks in place of ejected 2.5 disks. The capacity of the archive is doubled over time without the need to recopy old cases.

On-line case storage capacity can be increased and storage technology can be changed, if desired, by connecting additional archives to the server. Multiple archives, in different physical locations, might also be used to maintain a set of backup records. There is no need to use the same technology in all of the archives.

Interconnections

Clients and servers are interconnected using one of several available technical network architectures. Faster networks are usually more expensive. A prudent design provides enough speed to meet clinical needs with minimum surplus.

Hospitals often use Ethernet 10-base T connections. This provides a raw signaling rate of 10 megabits per second (effectively, a few uncompressed digital-cine frames per second). This is sufficient for simultaneous text communications between multiple users. Web-style video graphics need 100-base T Ethernet (100 megabits per second).

Achieving reasonable image transfer rates between a server and one client heavily loads a 100-base T line. A dedicated image network is required for

CV-PACS when Ethernet is used for the connections. Moving complete cases across the usual shared hospital network either will be unacceptably slow (normal transmission priority) or will temporarily block other network traffic (maximum priority).

The physical connection is either a copper wire or an optical fiber. High-quality copper wire is often used for 10- or 100-base T connections. Optical fiber has much more bandwidth capability than wire. The decision to use fiber or wire should be made after considering factors such as material and installation costs as well as possible future uses for the connection.

One or more hubs are used to connect clients and servers (Fig. 8-5). Hubs are standard network components. They are available in a range of bandwidths and connecting ports. Most hubs require external electrical power. Hubs need the same degree of UPS and emergency power protection, as do the servers.

To avoid traffic bottlenecks, high-volume imaging is usually handled on dedicated networks.

Image Workstations

The display workstation exists to deliver clinical images to the physician. The quality of these images is of paramount importance. Image quality is dependent on both workstation hardware and viewer software.

A "workstation" can be constructed from almost any off-the-shelf computer equipped with a CD drive or a network connection and public-domain viewing software. Such assemblies might be acceptable for casual use. They are unlikely to meet critical clinical performance requirements.

A computer acceptable to an adolescent for game play is powerful enough to use as the basis for a CV-PACS workstation. The presentation of real-time video gaming graphics from a CD demands the same system speed as that needed for cardiac cine. However, color requires greater bandwidth than gray scale.

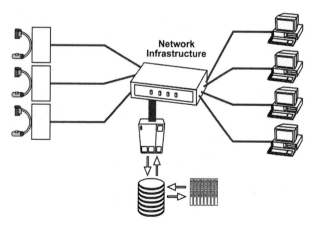

FIG. 8-5. **Network architecture for the client-server model.** The communications network is critical for departmental operations.

A few hardware enhancements are desirable. A PC configured to be used as an imaging workstation should have the maximum amount of RAM. This will maximize the number of immediately available images. It will also enhance the maximum available cine frame rate for looping and playback. Readily available internal hard disks can provide local storage for several studies.

Display workstations may require specialized video cards and monitor tubes. This is certainly true for those workstations used for primary diagnosis of chest radiographs. The need for specialized monitors is unclear for $512 \times 512 \times 8$-bit DICOM cardiac images. In some circumstances, the same monitors found in the interventional lab are needed in an image workstation. Individual evaluation, based on the local case mix, seems prudent.

SOFTWARE ESSENTIALS

Operating Systems

The Operating System (OS) is a layer of software functionally positioned between applications (e.g., word processor, cine viewer) and the workstation's hardware. An OS might exist in different versions so that it can run on different kinds of computer hardware (e.g., UNIX on Intel and Motorola processors). Different OSs may also be written to run on the same hardware (e.g., Windows 2000 and LINEX on an Intel processor). Application programmers usually use tools (software elements) built into the OS instead of coding everything from scratch.

A software application such as an image viewer is written to work with a specific operating system. This is not a problem if the workstation only runs one application. Desk space is finite and monitors are large. Ideally, the same workstation should be usable for all computerized tasks. However, few applications exist in versions compatible with most operating systems. Image-viewing software is a case in point. A "professional" OS provides performance-enhancing specialized tools. Consumer-oriented operating systems give the user greater flexibility in selecting software. The software designer must select an OS before coding a specific application. The network manager must decide whether to configure a workstation so that it can run one set of applications or another.

Viewing Software

Viewing hardware and software are critical parts of the clinical patient management chain.

The workstation exists to properly present images to the physician. This is the primary task of the viewing software. Secondary software tools provide means for case management and other functions.

Film is the traditional gold standard for image quality. In the past decade, many interventionalists have come to prefer the processed digital images seen in the lab. Consistently reproducing either image style (film or digital) is not trivial.

It is necessary to go back to imaging fundamentals. The brightness range at the output of the image intensifier depends on the interaction between the X-ray spectrum and the patient. The sensitometric properties of film govern the manner in which light intensity is converted into film blackening. The video camera [tube or charge-coupled device (CCD)] converts light into an electrical signal. These processes are nonlinear. Looking at a film on a monitor requires both the removal of electronic nonlinearity from the original video camera to the workstation monitor and the recreation of a sensitometric curve of a particular film.

Recreating the digital lab look includes the application of unsharp masking in the workstation. This is a computation-intensive process and requires a fast computer to obtain acceptable frame rates. For some workstations, the filter is applied to the images the first time that they are read from the CD or from the network. Processed images are stored in RAM. Replays from RAM are faster.

Optional public and private fields in the DICOM header give the cath lab's system means for transmitting image-processing parameters (e.g., look-up table and unsharp-mask filter) to the viewing software. The match between the interventional lab and the workstation is improved when viewing software uses this information.

MINI COURSE

Image and information workflow are necessary parts of any imaging department. Computers and networks should aid this process.

DICOM provides a framework for defining interoperability between hardware, software, and images.

Components need to be matched to medical requirements. This requires application-specific analysis.

9

Image Compression Methods in Digital Angiography

JACK T. CUSMA*

The replacement of cine film in the cardiac catheterization laboratory with digital imaging is difficult because of the large quantity of data required to represent and record a procedure. The technical requirements of digital cardiac angiography are demanding. The size of an exam record ranges from 500 megabytes (MB) to over 2000 MB or 2 gigabytes (GB). For a laboratory performing anywhere from 1000 to 10,000 procedures in a year, economical storage and reliable retrieval of procedure records remain significant challenges.

The real-time transfer of a fluoroscopic or cinefluorographic procedure requires a data bandwidth of 60 megabits per second (Mb/s) when using a small (512) matrix. However, even at that rate, large (1024) matrix images require four minutes to transfer every minute of recorded exam data. For comparison, the fast data connection available between many institutions is a T1 line (1.5 Mb/s data transfer rate). This connection uses forty minutes to transfer an examination that lasted only a minute.

At this time, *telemedicine* applications for remote consultation or access to exam results for referring physicians remain difficult to implement for dynamic angiographic sequences. Providing these services requires a reduction in the amount of transmitted data. It is not likely that there will be a reduction in the quantity of data required for accurate clinical decision making. Many applications are less demanding. The application of data compression methods to digital angiography is one way that the file sizes can be reduced to appropriately reasonable values.

---

*Mayo Foundation, Rochester, MN.

IMAGE COMPRESSION METHODS

Image compression algorithms are mathematical techniques for reducing the size of a file of digital data so that the resulting file still contains an acceptable portion of the original information content of the file. When an algorithm produces a file that can be restored to a form that is *identical* in every way to the original file, the compression method is referred to as *lossless* or *reversible*.

As an example, a medical image contains 512×512 pixels, each containing an intensity value ranging from 0 to 255. The size of the original file is 256 kilobytes (kB). This can be reversibly reduced to approximately 100 kB. The compression factor for this operation would be said to be $2.6:1$. When the compression is reversed, the result is a file that is again 256 kB in size in which each of the elements of that file matches one-by-one with the original file.

An alternative class of image compression results in greater degrees of reduction in the file size by not constraining the operation to being *completely* reversible. This class of *irreversible* or *lossy* compression methods results in a decompressed image in which the intensity at a particular image location may differ from the original image. This may lead to a perceptible difference in the way that the image appears to a user, for example, the physician reviewing the angiographic sequence.

Typically, lossy compression methods can be adjusted for different levels of "quality," trading off higher accuracy (similarity to the original image) in exchange for greater degrees of file reduction. In general, the greater the degree of compression, the more pronounced is the difference between the original and final images. Lossy compression can result in reductions in file sizes ranging from $5:1$ up to $100:1$. In the latter case, transmission of an image or an entire case could be achieved in 1/100th of the time that would have been required using the original images.

GENERAL COMPRESSION CONCEPTS

For any image data stored in a digital format (or for any type of data, for that matter), there is a varying degree of data *redundancy*. For example, a text file filled with the letter "a" repeated 1000 times requires 1000 bytes of storage space. It can be reversibly compressed by replacing the string of 1000 characters with a "code" of "1000a" so that the decompression process will recognize the code as an instruction to write out the letter "a" 1000 times. This code requires 5 bytes, resulting in a "compression ratio" of $200:1$.

In another example, a 512×512 image uniformly filled with the same gray level (e.g., 200) requires 262,144 bytes of uncompressed storage. A compression method represents the entire image as "200 512 512." Using the most compact available code, the image occupies only 5 bytes, resulting in a compression factor of over $50,000:1$.

Taking advantage of redundancies in data is the basis for all data compression methods. In some cases, a portion of the data storage capacity only records noise fluctuations. This clinically useless data can also be often discarded. The task, in selecting a compression method for application to medical images, is to determine what level of data can be removed without significantly impairing the information content.

The terms "visually" or "clinically" lossless refer to any compression method that does not affect the visual appearance or clinical utility of the image. In this context, one also needs to assess the environment in which the images are being displayed and observed because the *normal* viewing conditions will have an impact on whether a given solution is indeed visually lossless.

Most image compression methods can be described as a sequence of steps (Fig. 9-1). Every compression algorithm uses two or three of these steps. The first step in the process is a transformation or decomposition step in which the array of intensity values is converted to a representation that does not have as great a range as the original values. For example, in typical cardiac angiographic images, the intensity values can range from 0 to 255 (8 bit), 1023 (10 bit), or 4095 (12 bit), but their distribution in some alternative representation may not require as many different values. If properly chosen, this transformation will reduce redundancy and therefore result in a "spread" of values that is smaller than that in the original image, thereby requiring fewer bits of information for storage.

Another approach is to transform an image (or any type of information, for that matter) into a distribution of probabilities that a given value occurs. For example, an image containing 256 different intensity values would have

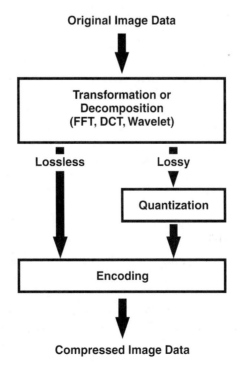

FIG. 9-1. Schematic diagram of the steps that comprise all data compression algorithms.

at most 256 different probabilities, but some values would occur much less frequently than others, some possibly not occurring at all, and this could be stored more efficiently.

The second step in the process depends on whether we are dealing with a reversible or nonreversible method. There is a quantization step in the nonreversible approach. This is where the lossy characteristic of these methods takes place. The process of quantization can be thought of as *smoothing* or "rounding off" the values produced in the transformation step. For example, the sequence of three numbers (213, 212, 218) can be rounded to 212, 212, 218 (the nearest even number). In this case, the number of bits required have been reduced from 8 (for 256 different values) to 7 required for the resulting 128 even numbers we have chosen to use. The lossy characteristic is obvious; we can no longer differentiate between the first two values in the trio, whereas, in the initial "image," there is a small difference between them.

The final step in the compression process is referred to as the *encoding* step; during this step, the resultant distribution of information from the previous step is stored in the most efficient way possible. If, for example, there are only 16 possible values resulting from the previous steps, it is much more efficient to store the distribution using 16 codes that correspond on a one-to-one basis with the values resulting from the transformation. Depending on the algorithm, a code table is then provided to the decompression process to facilitate the decoding of the compressed data.

LOSSLESS IMAGE COMPRESSION METHODS

In the ideal situation, the size of an image file would be reduced in such a manner that the reconstructed image result would be identical in every way to the original image acquired in the acquisition laboratory. There are many situations where one does not have the option of choosing between lossy and lossless compression methods. One cannot risk, for example, a change in even a single character or number because of the compression/decompression process for situations in which a long manuscript or a large set of research data is being transmitted or stored. A variety of lossless methods are in widespread general use, and some of these methods, or variations of them, are often applied to medical images.

Run-Length Encoding

Run-length encoding, or RLE, is one of the simplest forms of lossless data compression and can illustrate very basic concepts about how compression of files can occur. Essentially, the idea behind RLE is that, very often, the values in a large set—such as an image array of intensity values—occur in clusters or repeating patterns. In that case, efficiency results when the sequence (or array) of values is replaced with a new smaller sequence consisting of the value, followed by the number of times the value occurs in that string. Some simple examples of RLE were provided earlier in this chapter.

	Compressed Data	**Uncompressed Data**
Byte Data	08 16 00 04 17 21 19 22	16 16 16 16 16 16 16 16 17 21 19
Bit Data	10 13 04 ...	1111111110000000000001111

FIG. 9-2. Example of run length encoding. For strings with byte values (0–255) and for bit data (1, 0).

RLE is especially useful when one is dealing with just two values (e.g., 0 and 1). In this case, one could think of RLE as a replacement of alternating strings of ones and zeros with a number representing the value 1 or 0 and the number of times that each occur. The basic concept behind RLE is illustrated schematically in Figure 9-2.

The amount of compression that can be achieved using RLE on medical images is not as great as with other methods, but it is often used in combination with other methods. It is especially useful when an image contains large homogeneous areas such as a background mask set to the same value (all set to zero, for example).

RLE is frequently used in the compression of ultrasound images. It is one of the choices approved for compression of such images in the DICOM standard.

Huffman Coding

The method known as Huffman coding is an early development in data compression and represents the class of compression methods referred to as *variable-length* coding. This approach, in general, replaces values that occur most often in a source with shorter length "codes" and values that occur least frequently with longer length codes. Depending on the statistical distribution of values in an image, the resulting distribution of codes will have an average bit length smaller than that of the original distribution, which require a full 8 bits for every pixel value.

There are several approaches to Huffman encoding, depending on whether an assumed statistical distribution is used or whether the actual statistical distribution of values is calculated and a unique codebook is created for each image or set of images. In the former approach, a codebook would be created for digital coronary angiograms, and, every time a coronary angiographic image is processed, this codebook would be used to replace a particular pixel intensity with a code of varying length (in bits). The familiar Morse code is an example of a codebook specific to the occurrence of characters in the English language. A different codebook would be more efficient for compressing MRI scans (or Japanese characters).

In the second approach, the encoding process would be performed in two steps. First, the distribution of values would be determined for the image under consideration; next, a specific codebook mapping intensity values to codes would be generated. (The codebook for each image would be inserted into the header for that image.) Other, more efficient, encoding methods have been developed, but Huffman encoding remains widely used in combination with other methods. One example of interest is the lossless JPEG method, described below, which is used in the DICOM medium storage definition for cardiac X-ray angiographic images.

Ziv-Lempel Methods and Variations

In the description of the Huffman coding process, reference was made to the fact that its implementation was related to knowledge (or assumption) of the statistical probability of the occurrence of different input values. An alternative approach, known as dictionary-based compression, eliminates the need to know the probability distribution in the image. A dictionary is built from an input image, and, when a string of values in the image is recognized, it is replaced with the code value for it contained in the dictionary.

The origins of these techniques lie in the LZ77 algorithm, named after its inventors, Ziv and Lempel. The LZ77 algorithm is used in the popular PKZIP and WinZIP programs used in the distribution of files between computers. A variant, LZW compression, is used in the UNIX operating system. This algorithm is also used in the GIF image format found widely on the Internet and World Wide Web.

Differential Pulse Code Modulation

Regions within a medical image are fairly homogeneous (i.e., the values of pixels next to each other in the image are very similar). One method of compression, which takes advantage of this similarity, reduces the size of a file by replacing the original intensity values with the change in value from one pixel to the next. This method is an example of a predictive coding technique. Information about pixels that came before is used to predict the value of the pixels yet to come. Differential pulse-code modulation (DPCM) is one such method that reduces the range in intensity values in an image, thus, making it easy to compress.

JPEG

The JPEG image compression standard receives its name from the Joint Photographic Experts Group, the international standards group that developed and promoted the JPEG method for lossy image compression of photographic images. The JPEG standard also includes a lossless method that differs in many ways from the lossy algorithm. The lossless JPEG algorithm uses a combination of basic methods already described: a predictor stage similar to the DPCM method and a Huffman encoding step to take the difference values and replace them with codes that reduce the number of bits required to represent the pixels.

LOSSY COMPRESSION METHODS

Application of lossless compression methods to digital angiographic images typically results in data reduction on the order of about 3:1. Such degrees of compression are not enough to make a significant difference for many desired applications. For example, downloading of large image files through a telephone connection to the World Wide Web requires such long lengths of time that it cannot be pursued routinely. Reducing the size of these files so that they can be transmitted in a reasonable amount of time is a necessity for broadening access to image data.

Insertion of original images into a manuscript or presentation increases the size of the document by orders of magnitude compared with the space required if text alone were used. In many cases, a high amount of lossy compression can be tolerated with no loss in the value of the image for that specific application. (Most of the images in this book are actually compressed using lossy JPEG. Because of the subject matter, the images in Chapter 7 were compressed using lossless JPEG.) Many common desktop applications apply lossy methods to images without considering the effect on the information content of those images. For example, attachment of a medical image to an email letter about a patient's exam most certainly adds useful information to the textual summary. Image compression of 100:1 or greater is required for reasonable transmission time. The accompanying loss of clinical image quality may or may not be acceptable. Some of the more common lossy compression methods will be described below with a focus on the potential application of compression to digital cardiac angiography. This modality is emphasized in part because of the very large amounts of data required for recording of the clinical data and the dynamic nature of the recorded anatomic data.

Lossy JPEG

As noted above, the primary focus of the JPEG standards' effort was development of a standard method for lossy compression of still photographic images. In use since 1990, the JPEG algorithm remains one of the more widely available methods. It is a very successful exchange format and is often applied to medical image data.

The JPEG algorithm follows the general three-step approach illustrated in Figure 9-1. The transformation step in JPEG is performed using a mathematical procedure known as the discrete cosine transform (DCT). The process can be understood with a familiar example—a blood pressure waveform, which is a recording of the changes in pressure in time over the cardiac cycle. A transformation (Fourier transforms are typically used) converts the waveform to a representation in which the constituent frequencies are displayed. One can then see the relative contributions of higher frequencies compared with lower frequencies. Smoothing of the signal eliminates the higher frequency noise, making it easier to see the waveform shape information present in the lower frequencies.

Similar objectives are sought when applying the DCT to images; the major differences are of specifics rather than concepts. Rather than working with temporal frequencies (Hz) in an image, we are working with *spatial* frequencies [line pairs per mm (lp/mm)]. Very small objects such as stent struts and guide wires have higher frequency components, whereas large objects such as the diaphragm or lungs are largely low-frequency signals, except where an abrupt edge transition occurs. Because the image is a two-dimensional representation, the DCT produces information in two directions. The amplitude of a particular component represents how much of a contribution that frequency makes to the original image. As incorporated in JPEG, the DCT operation is applied to the image in 8-pixel by 8-pixel blocks. The image is broken up into such blocks, and operations are performed separately on these blocks. The origin of this requirement had to do with the relative computational efficiency rather than any physical justification. It is important to be aware of this aspect because it lies behind many of the artifacts that are apparent at high-compression ratios. Several of the steps involved are illustrated in Figure 9-3. After the DCT step, one has a new "image," which is also made up of the same number of corresponding 8 × 8 blocks. These blocks contain higher values in the

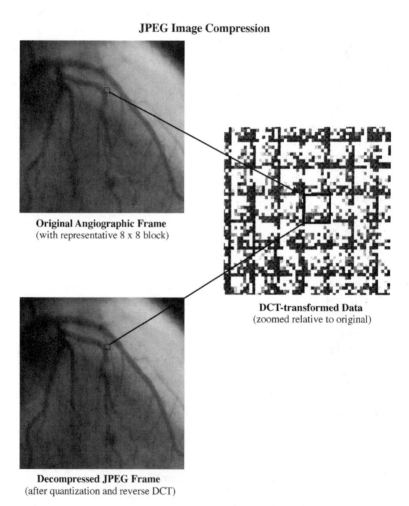

JPEG Image Compression

Original Angiographic Frame
(with representative 8 x 8 block)

DCT-transformed Data
(zoomed relative to original)

Decompressed JPEG Frame
(after quantization and reverse DCT)

FIG. 9-3. Illustration of the transformation process in JPEG. An 8 × 8 block in the original frame is transformed into frequency space using the DCT transform. After quantization, the DCT information is transformed to produce the 8 × 8 block of information in the decompressed image.

upper left-hand elements and very low values, including many zero values, as one moves down and to the right, where higher frequencies occur. To this point, this is a completely reversible process. The range of the information has been reduced by transforming to the frequency representation.

In the next step, referred to as the quantization step, we decide how much of the higher frequency information we "need" to represent the information in the image. This is somewhat analogous to application of a smoothing filter to a pressure waveform. The quantization process is just a truncation or "rounding" off the values in the DCT block. Depending on how much we round off, more or fewer of the elements become zero. This part of the process is where information is "lost." The remaining non-zero values representing relatively lower frequency information may or may not include *all* the information of interest. In JPEG nomenclature, a "quality factor" between 0 and 100 is selected, which leads to more or fewer zero elements in the DCT image. The use of the word "quality" is not to be interpreted as a reference to subjective image quality; that needs to be determined differently for every application and image type.

The final step in the JPEG process is to encode the quantized image using one or more lossless techniques. Depending on the original information in the image and the selected quality factor, compression ratios from 5:1 to 100:1 can be achieved.

The decompression process (Fig. 9-4) is a reversal of the compression steps. The algorithm operates on 8 × 8 blocks by unpacking the encoded zero and non-zero values, reversing the round-off quantization process, and inverting the DCT to go from the frequency to intensity representation. Figure 9-5 shows an example of a digital coronary angiographic frame that has undergone JPEG compression.

Two degradation effects can lead to visual artifacts in the final decompressed image. First, loss of high-frequency information may result in the loss of fine detail. Second, higher frequency information may be important in accurately reconstructing the transition between adjacent blocks. When this information is discarded by the quantization process, one gets abrupt changes at those edges where one 8 × 8 block meets another. This results in the "blocking" artifacts that are familiar to anyone who has received highly compressed images through email or through on-line services.

Motion JPEG

The JPEG standard described above was only designed for individual images. The technology has been extended to moving images (such as cardiac angiograms) using a straightforward approach known as motion JPEG (M-JPEG). In this method, each frame in a sequence of images is operated on individually,

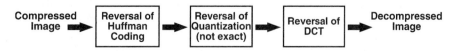

FIG. 9-4. Schematic diagram of the steps required to reverse the JPEG process.

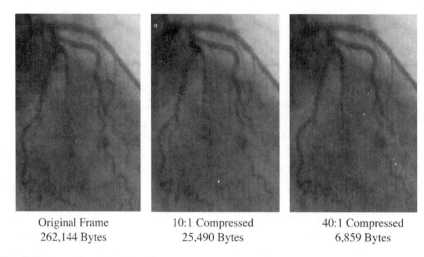

| Original Frame | 10:1 Compressed | 40:1 Compressed |
| 262,144 Bytes | 25,490 Bytes | 6,859 Bytes |

FIG. 9-5. Example of results of JPEG compression. The indicated file sizes refer to the entire frame, a portion of which is shown in the figure.

using the JPEG standard process. The compressed images are then combined sequentially into a single file. A table is usually added that lists the position of each individual frame within the file. This makes it easier to retrieve any individual frame without decompressing all the images. M-JPEG is found in many high-quality video-editing systems. These systems typically require fast computers or specialized hardware encoders to perform all the steps in the JPEG process in "real-time" on each new frame. It should be noted, however, that there is no official M-JPEG standard and interchange is not as reliable as with still JPEG images.

MPEG

A standard developed expressly to deal with moving pictures was published in 1992 by the Motion Picture Experts Group (MPEG). In general, MPEG and other methods intended for application to dynamic sequences of images take advantage of the similarity between successive images in a sequence. As in the previous discussion of redundancy within an image, most of the picture elements in an animated sequence such as a coronary angiogram or ultrasound exam change very little from one image to the next. Temporal compression methods take advantage of this relatively static situation, avoiding the necessity to repeat every value at every location. The difference between images for a picture element is coded and then decoded on the receiving end to reconstruct the original sequence.

The original MPEG-1 standard was capable of encoding incoming video streams at data rates of 1.5 Mb/s. This corresponds to sequences of 352 × 240 pixel color images displayed at 30 frames/s. MPEG-2 was released in 1993 to address the higher data rates required for digital transmission of broadcast television. The maximum data rate in MPEG-2, up to 9 Mb/s, accommodates processing of 720 × 480 color images at 30 frames/s. The MPEG-2 standard

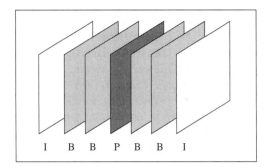

FIG. 9-6. Schematic diagram of the use of intra and interframe compression in MPEG. In common practice, the spacing between I-frames is 12 frames (0.4 seconds), and there are 3 P-frames and 8 B-frames in a "group-of-frames."

is used in the direct broadcast satellite systems as well as cable television systems. It is also the compression format used for DVD.

Image compression using MPEG has some similarities to the JPEG method. Some major differences can be illustrated with the help of Figure 9-6. Two types of compression are performed in MPEG: intraframe and interframe. Intraframe compression is performed on the contents of selected frames in a sequence. Application to these "I-frames" is essentially the same JPEG process described earlier. Interframe compression is used to encode the difference information between frames. It is performed by first decomposing each frame into 16×16 pixel blocks. The values in each "macroblock" are replaced with new values corresponding to the *difference* between the value in the frame and its predecessor. These difference values are then transformed using DCTs, quantized, and encoded. MPEG produces a high degree of compression by performing intraframe compression on only about 10% of the frames in a sequence with the remaining intermediate frames processed using the interframe encoding scheme. When there is little change in the scene from one frame to the next, many of the difference values for the macroblocks reduce to zero. The net result is a high compression ratio.

Because the MPEG standard is widely available, there is much interest in its use for dynamic medical images. In fact, there have been commercial offerings for both X-ray angiography and ultrasound imaging that store and transmit MPEG versions of the original streams. When considering the use of MPEG for such an application, it should be noted that random access to specific frames is limited. This means that, although one can display the moving sequence continuously, one cannot arbitrarily pause on a specific frame. This may not be acceptable for all clinical applications.

Wavelet Compression

JPEG and MPEG compression methods are widely available. Because they were not intended for medical images, it is not surprising that image degradation occurs that is not as acceptable in the medical application as in most consumer and publishing applications. One promising method that does not suffer the same degree of degradation is based on mathematical functions called wavelets. This method is called wavelet-based (or just wavelet) compression. This method seems to be the preferred compression method of the future. The general concepts behind wavelet compression are very similar to the three-step process illustrated earlier for JPEG. As with the DCT methods, a transformation is applied to the input image data in the first step. This time, the transformation is performed using a set of mathematical functions known as wavelets. The other major difference is that the transformation is applied to the entire image at once rather than to blocks of the image (Fig. 9-7). The result of transformation packs the information contained in the original image into a much narrower range of spatial frequencies so that it can be quantized and coded more efficiently (Fig. 9-8). There are a larger number of types of wavelet functions, permitting the selection of a family of functions that is best suited for a particular application. Transformation is followed by the now familiar steps of quantization and encoding. Wavelet quantization also causes irreversible data loss. There is less loss, however, than occurs using JPEG. An example of wavelet compression is shown in Figure 9-9.

The wavelet transformation is performed in several layers corresponding to increasingly higher spatial frequencies. This produces multiple versions of the image at one time. Successive versions are able to display higher frequencies (or smaller objects). Depending on the application, one varies the compression by "folding in" more of the higher frequency information.

Wavelet compression operates on the entire image at once. It does not produce the same edge artifacts found in block-based DCT methods. This permits a higher degree of compression without unacceptable image degradation.

JPEG2000

A draft of a proposed new standard, known as JPEG2000, was approved in late 1999. This is a revision of the JPEG standard reflecting advances in compression technology. Medical imaging requirements were specifically addressed in the development of the standard. It is likely that the deployment of this standard will have significant implications.

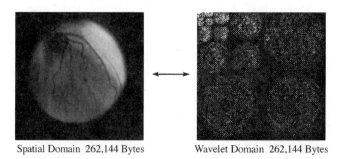

Spatial Domain 262,144 Bytes   Wavelet Domain 262,144 Bytes

FIG. 9-7. Illustration of the wavelet transformation. The image on the right represents the frequency information contained in the original image. Wavelet domain picture elements represent increasing frequency as they move down and away from the upper left-hand corner.

Energy Distribution for an XA Image After Wavelet Transform

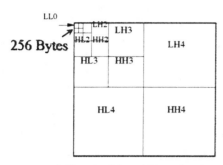
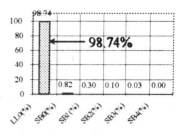

Subbands (5 Level Transform)   % Energy in Subbands for this XA image

FIG. 9-8. The distribution of information in the wavelet domain for the frame shown in Figure 9-7. The lowest frequency information, represented in the upper left-hand 256-byte block, contains over 98% of the information (energy) required to reconstruct the original frame.

IMAGE FORMATS

A degree of confusion exists between the compression algorithm used to reduce the size of an image file and the file format used to package or encapsulate the image file in a format that a reader or display program can deal with. Part of the confusion arises because specific compression methods are usually associated with a particular image format. One should think of a file format as the original information, along with a wrapper—header—which tells the receiver what kind of information is enclosed. As an example, one of the more familiar file formats is the tagged image file format or TIFF. In the TIFF format speci-

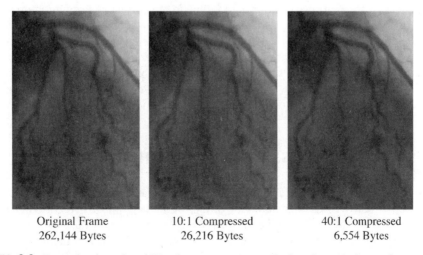

Original Frame   10:1 Compressed   40:1 Compressed
262,144 Bytes   26,216 Bytes   6,554 Bytes

FIG. 9-9. Example of results of Wavelet compression applied to the same frame shown in Figure 9-5. The indicated file sizes correspond to that required to store the complete frame.

fication, an image can be uncompressed (or raw) or can be converted using a variety of compression methods, including variations on RLE, Huffman Encoding, LZW, as well as lossless and lossy JPEG. The TIFF format specifies how a receiving display application is to recognize the type of compression; the viewer in use may or may not support that particular extension to TIFF. Another common file format, which incorporates compression, is GIF, which stands for the graphics interchange format, a popular file format for images that incorporates LZW data compression. A recently introduced file format for use on the World Wide Web is PNG for portable networks graphic format. The PNG format was developed, among other reasons, because use of the LZW algorithm in the GIF format is subject to royalties and an alternative was desired that was not so restricted. The compression algorithm in PNG is based on LZ77, together with Huffman coding.

COMPRESSION AND MEDICAL IMAGING STANDARDS

The DICOM (digital imaging and communications) standard provides a basic framework for medical imaging. DICOM defines standard formats for image storage and exchange.

Conformance to DICOM facilitates the exchange of images between different vendors. An important part of DICOM is the "conformance statement" describing an imaging component. Examination of the conformance statements of two components allows a determination as to their imaging compatibility.

DICOM permits the use of standard compression methods. A number of lossless methods are available, including lossless JPEG and RLE. To this point, only JPEG has been offered as an option for lossy compression. The encoding method used by the sender is identified so that the receiver can properly decode it. The required compression information is found in the DICOM image header.

A special note should be made regarding the use of compression methods in image storage data media such as cardiac angiography on recordable compact disks (CD-R). To date, the DICOM committee has only approved the use of lossless data compression. Individual vendors are permitted to add a second lossy version of the data on the DICOM CD. Although all conforming viewers must be able to display the standard lossless track, there is no assurance that any particular viewer can read the second lossy track.

EFFECTS OF COMPRESSION ON DIAGNOSTIC PERFORMANCE

The use of data compression in medical imaging became common practice early in the development of digital medical imaging technologies such as CT and MRI. Telemedicine requires significant compression to transfer images over standard telephone lines in a reasonable length of time. The nature of these images is such that a high degree of compression could be applied without degrading the clinical utility of the images for the specific application at hand.

As the range of applications increased, the question of the effects of image degradation on clinical decision-making resurfaced. This was an issue, for example, when the DICOM Working Group selected the acceptable options for the initial interchange media standard for cardiac angiography. In that situation, the task is the exchange of exam images between institutions for consultation and planning of additional procedures. Because of the clinical importance of that application, priority was placed on maintaining the highest image quality, identical to that available at the time of image acquisition.

The decision to use lossy image compression in any clinical application requires determination of the effects of the compression on the user's ability to extract the required clinical information. There have been a number of approaches: for the purposes of this chapter, we will focus on those that have addressed the issue of dynamic cardiac X-ray images acquired in a digital format. The studies that have been performed can be grouped into two classes: (i) those that assessed the effects of compression on the visual performance of clinical observers; (ii) those that investigated the effect of compression on quantitative measurements such as quantitative coronary arteriography (QCA) from images. Among the second group, there were a number that indicated that significant differences begin to occur in computerized measurements of stenosis severity at compression levels on the order of 12:1 to 15:1. These results are important for consideration of whether compressed images should be archived for long-term storage and whether they should be used for clinical trials incorporating the use of QCA measurements.

A multicenter study was designed and performed in the late 1990s (by ACC, ESC, and the DICOM committee) to evaluate the effects of lossy compression on both visual performance and quantitative measurements. This study collected image data from multiple laboratories around the world representing a variety of digital angiography equipment and performed visual assessment studies using experienced angiographers from multiple laboratories.

In Phase I of the study, observers were shown sequences of images in a blinded fashion and were asked to identify clinical features of interest such as calcium, dissections, stents, and so forth, as well as to assess the severity of specified stenoses. Their findings were compared with the answers found by a panel of experts working with the original uncompressed image data. The results indicated that degradation of performance begins to take place at a level of 10:1 lossy JPEG compression.

In Phase II, a different group of observers was shown pairs of image sequences side-by-side on a single workstation; they were asked whether they could detect a difference between the sequences. The results of this more stringent test agreed with the first phase that degradation in clinical performance begins at around 10:1.

In Phase III, the effect on QCA measurements was determined using a subset of angiographic frames taken from the complete set used for the first two phases. Here, as well, compression at 10:1 resulted in measurement variability that was deemed unacceptable. It should be noted that these results were only valid for lossy JPEG compression using standard methods; any other compression method under consideration for clinical applications should be evaluated using similar methodology.

SUMMARY

There are many applications for which reduction in the volume of data is desired. Clinical users should be aware of the potential effects of compression schemes on their images and should make every effort to avoid excessive degradation for the application of interest.

Compression techniques facilitate rapid and widespread image distribution. This is a desirable objective and is important for patient care. However, the appropriate quality image needs to be delivered to each clinical user. Following the procedures recommended by professional societies and standards bodies is advised.

10

Quantitative Coronary Arteriography

JOHAN H.C. REIBER,[1,2,3] GERHARD KONING,[1] JOAN C. TUINENBURG,[1] and
BOB GOEDHART[1]

INTRODUCTION

The dynamics of coronary atherosclerosis, that is progression and regression of
coronary atherosclerotic lesions, the healing of lesions, and the development
of new ones, have intrigued cardiologists since the time that this process could
be followed by repeated coronary arteriographic X-ray examinations.

A complicating factor in the evaluation of the severity and extent of the
degree of coronary atherosclerosis is the occurrence of compensatory mechanisms, which is nowadays denoted by the term coronary artery remodeling.
Glagov et al were the first to describe that compensatory enlargement of the
human atherosclerotic coronary arteries occurs during the early stages of plaque
formation. This compensatory enlargement results in the preservation of a
nearly normal lumen cross-sectional area so that an atherosclerotic plaque will
have less hemodynamic effects. This "outward" growth process stops at a certain point in time as it reaches the maximal stretching capacities of the vessel,
followed by subsequent further "inward" growth of the plaque. Once the lumen
of the vessel becomes impaired, it becomes visible by X-ray arteriography,
which is a two-dimensional projection technique, allowing only the visualization of the contrast-filled lumen.

Usually, atherosclerosis is present as a focal narrowing over a limited
length, superimposed on a diffuse atherosclerotic process within the entire
artery. Because X-ray arteriography only depicts the remaining opening of an
artery, it underestimates the presence of diffuse atherosclerosis and is unable

Departments of [1]Radiology and [2]Cardiology, Leiden University Medical Center, and [3]Interuniversity
Cardiology Institute of the Netherlands, Utrecht, The Netherlands.

to detect the early stages of coronary atherosclerosis. Until today, cross-sectional imaging of the individual coronary arteries and the assessment of the arterial wall have been the exclusive domain of intravascular ultrasound (IVUS). IVUS is able to provide real-time high-resolution tomographic images of sections of the arterial wall and to demonstrate the presence or absence of compensatory arterial enlargement.

The purely visual interpretation of images is subjective and therefore associated with significant inter- and intra-observer variations. There has been a continuing interest in developing robust and automated segmentation techniques to obtain objective and reproducible data from cardiac angiograms. In the late 1970s, quantitative coronary arteriography (QCA) was developed to quantify vessel motion and the effects of drugs on the regression and progression of coronary artery disease. So far, QCA has been the only technique that allows the accurate and reliable assessment of the morphological changes within the entire coronary vasculature over time (regression/progression studies). For single, individual coronary segments, quantitative coronary ultrasound (QCU) is also gaining interest. In interventional cardiology, QCA is widely used for vessel sizing and the assessment of the efficacy of the individual procedures, as well as in core laboratories to study the efficacy of these procedures in large patient populations.

The goal of this chapter is to provide an overview of the current approaches to quantitative image analyses that use automated edge detection techniques in the field of quantitative coronary arteriography.

ANALOG OR DIGITAL IMAGE ACQUISITION AND ANALYSIS

Let us first describe the differences between the cine film and digital techniques in the image acquisition and analysis portions of the X-ray imaging chains (Fig. 10-1). For QCA purposes, the cine film is mounted on a cine-video converter, which features optical magnification and an analog or digital video camera for conversion of the images into video format. The converters must

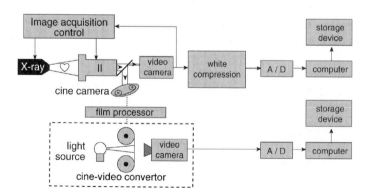

FIG. 10-1. Block diagram of combined film-based and digital angiographic system.

satisfy specific requirements for QCA applications, such as zooming capabilities (minimally 1- to 3-fold continuous), high spatial resolution of the optical chain, even brightness distribution over the field-of-view, high quality of the video camera, and so forth. To analyze a selected coronary segment, a region of interest (ROI) encompassing the coronary segment or catheter is magnified optically approximately 2.3-fold, such that pixel sizes in the range of 0.08–0.10 mm are obtained after digitization; this range of pixel sizes has been found to be optimal for our contour detection approaches. The video signal from the camera in the cine-film projector is digitized, e.g. at a resolution of 512×512-pixels $\times$ 8 bits, and stored in the workstation for subsequent analysis.

In the digital approach, the output image of the image intensifier is projected onto the input target of a video camera. The analog video output signal is modified electronically in the so-called "white compression" unit, resulting in greater contrast differences in the parts with high X-ray absorption (e.g. vertebrae and contrast filled arteries or the ventricle) and lower contrast differences in the areas with low X-ray absorption (e.g. lung area). This markedly improves the image quality of the images. Next, the resulting video signal is digitized at a resolution of 512×512 pixels $\times$ 8 bits on most X-ray systems or up to 1024×1024 pixels $\times$ 12 bits on some other X-ray systems and stored on the high-speed disks of the digital imaging system for subsequent review and possibly quantitative analysis. Because optical magnification is not possible in this approach, the pixel size in the standard $512 \times 512 \times 8$ bits mode will be markedly larger than achievable with the cine film. An entire patient study can be stored in DICOM format on CD-R after the procedure.

From the user's point of view, the analysis of digital images on the QCA workstation is similar to the analysis of cine-film frames. However, there are a number of important differences between cine film and digital media:

- Cine film has a nonlinear density function (H&D curve), which differs between hospitals and which may differ slightly from day to day or week to week. Digital systems are characterized by well-defined nonlinear functions (the white compression).

- Cine film is hampered by film grain noise, which is absent on the digital systems.

- On cine film, the vessels are visible as bright structures on a dark background; in the digital images, they are dark structures on a bright background.

- Edge enhancement is not possible on cine film. It is frequently used on digital images.

The QCA algorithms must be optimized for the image medium to take care of all these differences listed above. One cannot just apply first- and second-derivative functions (the kernels) derived for cine-film applications to a digital image without modifications and expect the same systematic and random errors.

BRIEF HISTORY OF QUANTITATIVE CORONARY ARTERIOGRAPHY

Since the first papers on QCA were published in 1977 and 1978, this field has grown substantially. First-generation QCA systems, developed in the 1980s, were based on 35-mm cine-film analysis. Second-generation systems (1990–1994) were characterized by further improvements in the quality of the edge detection, often applied to digital images, and included corrections for the overestimation of the vessel sizes below approximately 1.2 mm. It should be noted that the edge-detection algorithm for the cine-film analysis cannot simply be applied to digital images, which have other image characteristics; therefore, digital images require further tuning of these algorithms. Third-generation (1995–1998) QCA systems provided solutions for the quantitative analysis of complex lesion morphology using, for example, the Gradient Field Transform (GFT®) and improved diameter function calculations. With the establishment of DICOM for digital image exchange and HL7 for administrative data, the need for integration of QCA systems into the complex environment of the hospital was recognized. Finally, with the greatly enhanced capabilities of modern workstations, fourth-generation QCA systems have been available since 1999; these systems are characterized by simplified portability to digital DICOM viewers, network connectivity, and improved reporting and database facilities. Although most modern QCA packages are based on the linear programming approach for contour detection, there are still differences in the qualities of these packages, which need to be documented by extensive validation reports.

BASIC PRINCIPLES OF QUANTITATIVE CORONARY ARTERIOGRAPHY

Requirements for QCA

For a QCA package to be applicable in a routine clinical or research environment, a number of requirements must be met:

- It must require minimal user interaction in the selection and processing of the coronary segment to be analyzed.
- It should require minimal editing of the automatically determined results. The user should seldom feel the need to edit the intermediary results, such as the detected contours of the arterial segments.
- It should have a short analysis time, on the order of 10 seconds or less.
- It should provide highly accurate and precise results, in other words, small systematic and random errors, respectively, in the assessment of the morphological data. This should be demonstrated by extensive validation studies using phantom and routinely acquired clinical studies.

Basic Principles of Automated Contour Detection

The general principles and characteristics of a modern QCA software package that satisfies these requirements can best be illustrated by the QCA-CMS®

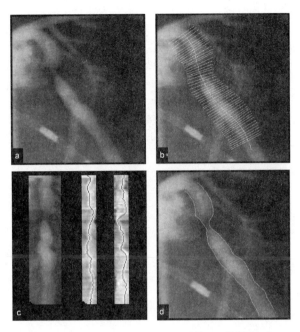

FIG. 10-2. Basic principles of the minimum cost analysis (MCA) contour-detection algorithm. a: Initial segment. b: Scanlines defined. c: Straightened for analysis; contours calculated. d: Contours returned to initial image; diameter measurements performed.

(Cardiovascular Measurement System, MEDIS[4]) algorithms developed in our laboratory.

The QCA operator selects in the ROI (Fig. 10-2a) the coronary segment to be analyzed by using the computer mouse to define the start and end points of that segment. Next, an arterial pathline through the segment of interest is computed automatically (Fig. 10-2b).

The contour-detection procedure is carried out in two iterations relative to a model. In the first iteration, the detected pathline is the model. To detect the contours, scanlines are defined perpendicular to the model (Fig. 10-2b). For each point or pixel along such a scanline, the corresponding edge-strength value (local change in brightness level) is computed as the weighted sum of the corresponding values of the first- and second-derivative functions applied to the brightness values along these scanlines (Fig. 10-3). The resulting edge-strength values are input to the so-called minimal cost analysis (MCA) contour-detection algorithm, which searches for an optimal contour path along the entire segment (Fig. 10-2c). The individual left and right vessel contours detected in the first iteration now serve as models in the second iteration, in which the MCA contour-detection procedure is repeated relative to the new models.

To correct for the limited resolution of the entire X-ray system, the MCA algorithm is modified in the second iteration based on an analysis of the quality

---

[4]MEDIS medical imaging systems, Leiden, The Netherlands.

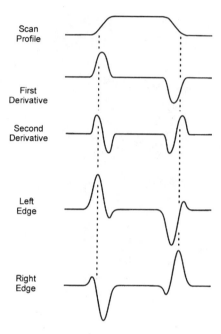

FIG. 10-3. Schematic presentation of the brightness profile of an arterial vessel assessed along a scanline perpendicular to the local pathline direction and the computed 1st-derivative, 2nd-derivative, and the combinations of these 1st- and 2nd-derivative function; the maximal values of the last functions determine the edge positions.

of the imaging chain in terms of its resolution, which is of particular importance for the accurate measurement of small diameters, as in coronary obstructions. If such a correction is not applied, significant overestimation of vessel sizes below approximately 1.2 mm would occur. In the literature, other approaches have been described as well.

If the QCA operator does not agree with one or more parts of the detected contours, they can be edited in various ways. However, each manual editing is followed by a local MCA iteration, so that the newly detected contours are truly based on the local brightness information. In other words, the operator indicates roughly where the contour should be detected, and the MCA algorithm searches for the final contour based on the available image information (Fig. 10-2d). The MCA approach has been demonstrated to be very robust.

Calibration Procedure

Calibration of the image data is performed on a nontapering portion of a contrast-filled catheter using an MCA edge-detection procedure similar to that applied to the arterial segment. In this case, however, additional information is used in the edge-detection process because this part of the catheter is known to be characterized by parallel boundaries. It should also be recognized that the catheter calibration procedure is the weakest link in the analysis chain because of the variable image quality of the displayed catheters. Another potential problem with calibration is the out-of-plane magnification, which occurs when the catheter and the coronary segment are positioned at different distances from the image intensifier. Biplane calibration could overcome this problem but is rarely applied in routine QCA. A number of recommendations for catheter calibration are reviewed in the section *Guidelines for Catheter Calibration*.

Coronary Segment Analysis

From the left- and right-hand contours of the arterial segment, a diameter function is determined (Fig. 10-4). It must be stressed that the calculation of the width of a vessel segment along its trajectory from proximal to distal, resulting in a diameter function, is not a trivial task, certainly not in a situation of complex anatomy. In X-ray imaging, pincushion distortion caused by the convex input screen of the image intensifier may be present, which may influence the diameter calculations. Correction for this distortion should not be applied in routine single-plane QCA, as this may introduce more artifacts rather than resolve problems.

The most widely used parameter to describe the severity of a coronary obstruction is the percentage of diameter narrowing. Calculation of this parameter requires that a reference diameter value be computed, for which two options are available: 1) a user-defined reference diameter as positioned by the user at a so-called "normal" portion of the vessel and 2) the automated or interpolated reference diameter value. In practice, this last approach is preferred because it requires no user interaction and takes care of any tapering of the vessel. For that purpose, a reference diameter function is calculated by an iterative regression technique and displayed in the diameter function as a

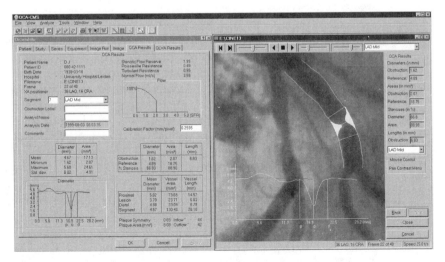

FIG. 10-4. The results of the minimal cost analysis, including the reconstructed original vessel contours, plaque area (shaded), and the diameter function, are presented for QCA-CMS V4.0. All the derived absolute and relative QCA parameters are presented in the QCA DICOM-box (*left*).

straight line. The iterative approach has been used to exclude the influence of any obstruction or ectatic area as much as possible, so that it represents a best approximation of the vessel size before the occurrence of the focal narrowing. Now that the reference diameter function is known, reference contours can be reconstructed around the actual vessel segment, representing the original size and shape of the vessel before the focal disease occurred. However, the possible presence of any diffuse atherosclerosis cannot be corrected for. Finally, the difference in area between the detected lumen contours and the reference contours is a measure for the atherosclerotic plaque in this particular angiographic view and is shaded in Figure 10-4.

The actual reference diameter value corresponding with a selected obstruction is now taken as the value of the reference diameter function at the site of the obstruction, so that neither overestimation nor underestimation occurs. From the reference diameter value and the obstruction diameter, the percent diameter narrowing is calculated. This automated approach has been found to be very reproducible.

The Flagging Procedure

In the majority of QCA analyses, the calculation of the reference diameter function and the reconstruction of the reference contours provide a reliable representation of the vessel segment. However, over-dilated stents, vessels with extremely ectatic areas, overlap of vessel segments, and so forth, negatively influence the calculation of the reference diameter function. This is illustrated in Figure 10-5a: The ectatic area proximal to the obstruction results in a significant tapering of the reference diameter function, such that the normal vessel size would not be measured correctly. In this case, a stenosis of 71% would be measured (obstruction diameter of 1.23 mm, reference diameter of 4.35 mm); this is a very undesirable situation. Therefore, another option being the "flagging" procedure has been implemented. The user can "flag" the portion of the vessel segment (in Fig. 10-5b, the proximal portion of the vessel), and the corresponding diameter values are excluded in the subsequent calculation of the reference diameter function. The correctly calculated reference diameter function and reconstructed reference contours are presented in Figure 10-5b, which is more in line with what one would expect. For this case, a narrowing of 67% (obstruction diameter of 1.23 mm, reference diameter of 3.78 mm) is measured.

From the calculated diameter function, many parameters are derived automatically, including the site of maximal percentage of stenosis, the obstruction diameter, the corresponding automatically determined reference diameter, and the extent of the obstruction. Additionally derived parameters include obstruction symmetry, inflow and outflow angles, the area of the atherosclerotic plaque, and functional information, such as the stenotic flow reserve or SFR. The SFR describes, on the basis of a mathematical/physiological model, how much the flow can possibly increase under maximal hyperemic conditions in that particular coronary segment due to that single obstruction; it can also be described as a wind tunnel test of that stenosis under standardized conditions

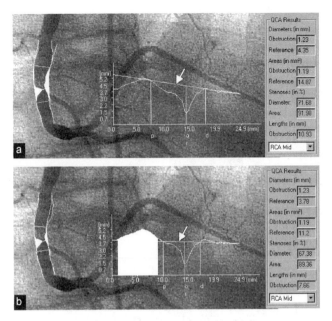

FIG. 10-5. **Example of a vessel with an ectatic area.** a: Straightforward application of the reference diameter function would lead to arbitrary, erroneous results, in this case in significant tapering of the reference diameter function (arrow). b: By "flagging" the proximal ectatic area, a nontapering reference diameter function (arrow) results and appropriately reconstructed vessel reference contours.

(Fig. 10-4). In a disease-free segment, the SFR equals 4–5, a value that decreases as the severity of the obstruction increases.

Complex Vessel Morphology

As explained earlier, modern contour-detection approaches are based on the MCA algorithm, which has been demonstrated to be fast and robust for images that may vary significantly in image quality. This approach has been shown to work very well as long as the vessel outlines are relatively smooth in shape. However, complex vessel morphology may occur after coronary intervention (e.g. when a dissection occurs).

In its design, the MCA technique is hampered when tracing very irregular and complex boundaries. First, the algorithm can select only one point per scanline. However, when the coronary artery has irregular boundaries, for example, at a complex lesion, this condition may not be satisfied (Fig. 10-6). Second, the edge strength or derivative values are calculated only along the direction of the scanlines, whereas the highest edge strength values may occur in other directions. Third, the results are therefore highly dependent on the actual directions of these scanlines; a slight change in direction may result in other contour points. To circumvent these problems and limitations, and as a result be able to adequately analyze such very irregular stenoses, we developed

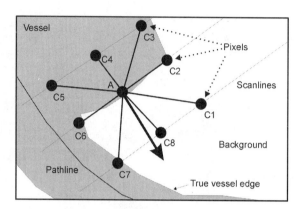

FIG. 10-6. Schematic representation of a vessel with its pathline, the scanlines, and the search directions for the GFT® algorithm.

a new algorithm, the Gradient Field Transform (GFT®), which will be illustrated with the graphical example given in Figure 10-6.

Scanlines are defined perpendicular to the pathline as in standard MCA. The closed circles in Figure 10-6 represent pixels along the scanlines. Pixel A is a contour point under consideration. In search for the next point of the arterial boundary, the MCA algorithm would only consider points C7, C8, and C1. Contrary to that, the GFT algorithm takes all of its eight neighboring points (C1–C8) into account. Each branch from a particular scan point to a neighboring scan point is assigned a different cost value (a mathematical technique), which is a function of its edge strength and the angle between the direction of the edge and the direction of the branch. The goal of the algorithm now is to find an optimal path between one node on the first scanline of the vessel segment and one node on the last scanline of this segment.

In practice, the entire contour detection procedure is applied twice to a coronary segment: the first time the detected pathline is used as a model and the GFT is carried out. In the second iteration, the initially detected contours are again used as models for the subsequent detection of the arterial boundaries, this time using the standard MCA algorithm. This approach enables the GFT to follow more irregular arterial boundaries and even follow reversal of the contour direction, for example, to follow flaps. An illustrative example of the GFT is given in Figure 10-7.

The obstruction diameters of complex lesions assessed by GFT analysis are, on the average, 0.25 mm smaller than those detected by the MCA algorithm. The detected contours are a little more irregular because the algorithm is more sensitive to noise in all possible spatial directions. However, we believe that these data represent a correct reflection of the vessel's morphology. These irregularities may also provide prognostic information. This is a subject that needs to be investigated in future studies.

Our experiences with GFT analyses indicate that this approach is recommended for the analysis of ostial lesions and of radiopaque stents. With the appropriate optical zooming (in an off-line configuration), GFT analysis is able

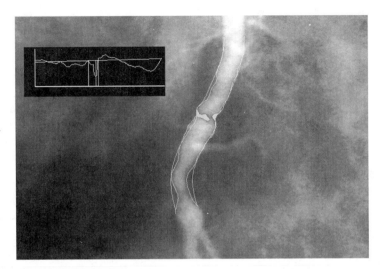

FIG. 10-7. Example of outcome of GFT analysis on a vessel segment with very severe complex stenosis. Conventional approaches with the MCA algorithm are not able to follow automatically the abrupt changes in morphology.

to follow the outer boundaries of the stent struts and the contrast lumen in between the stent struts.

Densitometry

Because the X-ray arteriogram is a two-dimensional projection image of a three-dimensional structure, measured vessel sizes may be of limited value in vessels with very irregular cross sections. For many years, great efforts have been devoted in trying to derive from the brightness levels within the coronary arteries information about the path lengths of the X-rays through these vessels. If such a relationship could be established, one would obtain the information required to compute the cross-sectional areas from a single angiographic view. This approach is called the densitometric measurement technique.

Theoretically, densitometry would seem the ultimate solution for the computation of the vessel's cross-sectional area from a single angiographic view. However, so far, densitometry has not provided reliable results, particularly from cine film, and, as a result, the interest in it has largely diminished. It may be of interest to revisit the densitometric approaches for the digital systems in which the entire transfer function of the X-ray system is better controlled and more stable than with the use of cine film. However, other potential error sources remain.

GUIDELINES

Guidelines for Catheter Calibration

For an automated edge detection of the catheter shaft or tip to be reliable, it is necessary that the image contrast of the catheter and the sharpness of the edges be sufficiently high. For that purpose, restrictions have been formulated as to the size and the types of the catheters, resulting in so-called QCA-approved catheters.

An important issue has always been whether the catheter should be flushed or contrast filled for the calibration procedure. From our observations and validation studies, we have concluded that it is recommended that contrast-filled catheters of the exact same type (size, material, and manufacturer) be used for both baseline and follow-up measurements.

Guidelines for QCA Acquisition Procedures

The primary objective of QCA measurements in clinical trials is to allow more precise and reliable analyses of the real changes after interventions, namely, acute lumen gain and late lumen loss expressed in millimeters. This is best achieved when exactly the same setting is applied during the procedure and at the follow-up studies, that is, replication of same views, same doses of intracoronary nitroglycerin, same contrast media, same catheter type or material, and, if feasible, same catheterization room.

QCA VALIDATION

Whichever QCA analytical software package is being used, it will always produce numbers describing the morphology of the coronary segment analyzed. However, validation studies must demonstrate the true strengths and weaknesses, as well as the clinical validity, of such analytical package.

It has been well accepted that the results from validation studies should be described in terms of the systematic error or accuracy, defined by the average signed difference between the corresponding measurements (i.e., *measurement 1* minus *measurement 2*), and the random error or precision, defined by the standard deviation of these signed differences.

For a QCA technique to be acceptable, guidelines for systematic and random error values of absolute vessel dimensions have been established. These guidelines are shown in Table 10-1; the systematic error values for the Plexiglass phantom apply to each of the individual measurements.

Plexiglass Phantom Studies

The latest QCA-CMS V4.0 analytical package was validated using a Plexiglass phantom with tube sizes in the range of 0.80–5.00 mm. The tubes were filled with 100% contrast medium and positioned such that they were approximately horizontal and vertical on the images. Data was obtained at 60, 75, and 90 kV, using both 5-in. and 7-in. image intensifier sizes. Three different analyses were carried out: 1) off-line from 35-mm cine film, 2) off-line from DICOM-CD, and 3) on-line from video digitized frames. The results are presented in Table 10-2.

The data from Table 10-2 can be summarized as follows: Both systematic and random errors were within the guidelines for all three acquisition modes.

TABLE 10-1. Guidelines for systematic and random errors of a state-of-the-art QCA System

	Systematic error (mm)	Random error (mm)
Plexiglass phantom		
Off patient	<0.10	0.10–0.13
On patient	<0.10	0.10–0.13
In vivo study		0.10–0.20
Postmortem study		0.20–0.30
Inter/intra-observer variabilities		0.10–0.15
Short-term variabilities		0.15–0.25
Medium-term variabilities		0.20–0.30
Long-term variabilities		0.20–0.30

Variability or random errors increased with increasing kilovolt level due to the decreasing image contrast levels. The lowest variability was obtained with the digital 512^2 images (although the differences are small). The overall variability was found to be slightly higher when the phantom was positioned on a patient's chest compared with an off-patient situation (data not presented here).

In Vivo Plexiglas Plugs

The ultimate test for a QCA system is the analysis of clinical images of obstructions with known dimensions. For this purpose, small Plexiglass plugs (outer diameters: of 2.5–3.5 mm, inner diameters of 0.5–1.57 mm, length of approximately 7.5 mm) were introduced with a catheter into the coronary arteries of dogs. Images were acquired on cine film, as well as in digital format. From the obstructive region, the mean diameter and the standard deviation of the diameter measurements were assessed; the mean diameter was compared with the known true inner diameter of the plug. Systematic and random errors were of the same magnitude as the results from the coronary phantom on a homogenous background and on patient anatomy.

TABLE 10-2. QCA-results for a Plexiglass phantom acquired on a homogeneous background

II-Size	kV-Level	Digital 512 S.E. ± R.E.	On-Line S.E. ± R.E.	Cinefilm V4.0 S.E. ± R.E.
5″	60 kV	0.00 ± 0.04	−0.02 ± 0.05	0.03 ± 0.03
	75 kV	0.00 ± 0.07	−0.02 ± 0.07	−0.02 ± 0.07
	90 kV	−0.01 ± 0.09	−0.04 ± 0.11	−0.04 ± 0.11
7″	60 kV	0.01 ± 0.05	0.00 ± 0.05	0.05 ± 0.05
	75 kV	0.01 ± 0.07	−0.02 ± 0.08	0.00 ± 0.08
	90 kV	−0.01 ± 0.10	0.00 ± 0.10	−0.03 ± 0.10

Abbr.: S.E. = Systematic Error, R.E. = Random Error.

TABLE 10-3. Inter- and intra-observer and short- and medium-term variabilities using the ACA/DCI V1.0 analytical software package

Variabilities	Obstruction diameter (mm) S.E. ± R.E.	Reference diameter (mm) S.E. ± R.E.
Inter-observer	−0.02 ± 0.11	−0.01 ± 0.13
Intra-observer	0.03 ± 0.10	0.03 ± 0.13
Short-term	0.00 ± 0.19	−0.02 ± 0.22
Medium-term	0.03 ± 0.18	−0.02 ± 0.34

Abbr.: S.E. = Systematic Error, R.E. = Random Error.

Inter- and Intra-Observer and Short- and Medium-Term Variabilities

Extensive data on inter- and intra-observers and on short- and medium-term variabilities are available. A summary of these results using the ACA/DCI[5] V1.0 analytical software package is presented in Table 10-3. The inter- and intra-observer variability studies on a set of routinely obtained digital coronary arteriograms demonstrated that the systematic errors were approximately zero; in other words, no systematic differences were found. The random errors for the obstruction diameter were less than 0.11 mm, and, for the interpolated reference diameter, these were less than 0.13 mm. Larger variabilities were observed when the study was extended to so-called "short-term" investigations, with repeated angiographic acquisition after 5 minutes, and "medium-term" investigations, with repeated acquisitions at the end of the catheterization procedure under standardized circumstances. These larger variabilities can be explained mainly from variations in the repeated calibration procedures based on the catheter.

Inter-Laboratory Variability

With the widespread use of QCA in different laboratories, the question comes up of how well the results from these QCA laboratories correlate. This is of particular relevance for core laboratories, which at a certain point in time may wish to combine their QCA data from similar trials for meta-analysis purposes or otherwise want to compare data, for example, from angiographic procedures, carried out in different countries. Systematic differences most likely exist in the absolute dimensions between the two laboratories. Hopefully, the two laboratories show the same trends between baseline and follow-up studies. However, these assumptions cannot be taken for granted. Validation studies need to be carried out to demonstrate the differences in an objective manner.

If two laboratories use the same equipment, differences will exist in the image quality of the coronary arteriograms; in the way the angiograms are analyzed in terms of the frame selection, frame digitization (for cine film), and the definition of the coronary segments; in the experience of the technicians in the actual analysis of the images. Studies have clearly demonstrated that

[5]Philips Medical Systems, Best, The Netherlands.

TABLE 10-4. Inter-laboratory systematic and random errors in the individual measurements for two highly standardized and collaborating core labs

N = 63	Systematic error	Random error
Obstruction diameter (mm)	−0.06	0.14
Reference diameter (mm)	−0.02	0.15
Percentage diameter stenosis (%)	1.83	4.96
Mean segment diameter (mm)	0.00	0.10

significant analysis differences may occur between different angiographic core laboratories, particularly when different QCA systems are used.

Two core laboratories (Heart Core bv in Leiden, the Netherlands, and the Montreal Heart Institute in Montreal, Canada) have standardized their entire QCA procedure. The errors between the two sites for the most important QCA parameters are given in Table 10-4. These data indicate that the systematic errors between the two sites are very small and that the random errors are within ranges similar to earlier reported inter-observer variabilities (Table 10-3). It should be noted that an additional potential error source is the different video systems on the cine-film digitizers (PAL and NTSC) used by the two sites. From this study, it can be concluded that interlaboratory variabilities between highly organized and standardized QCA core labs can be in the same range as the reported inter- and intra-observer variabilities. Furthermore, it is clear that regular testing of the entire analysis procedure is necessary to remain within the standards that have been set.

Concluding Remarks

With an analysis time of less than 10 seconds, efficient tools are now available for the objective and reproducible assessment of the coronary arteries and the changes resulting from intervention procedures. Our validation studies indicate that cine-film analysis is associated with a slightly smaller random error (by 10–15%) than by the digital analysis. The performance of a modern QCA workstation like the QCA-CMS system is such that the computer is not the limiting factor in such applications. Items such as frame selection, documentation of the results, and so forth now occupy most of the time.

APPLICATIONS OF QCA: OFF-LINE AND ON-LINE

In the new digital or DICOM era, QCA is clearly used in different ways, which we will refer to for reasons of simplification by the notations "off-line QCA" and "on-line QCA."

By off-line QCA, we mean one or more QCA workstations that are not directly connected to the image-generating X-ray system in the catheterization laboratories. Furthermore, it is possible that multiple QCA workstations are

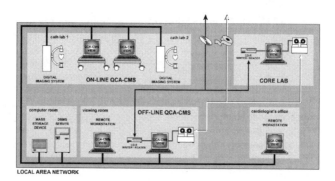

FIG. 10-8. Schematic diagram of off-line and on-line applications of QCA workstations.

connected to an internal network to exchange image data with a file server for central storage purposes.

Typical applications for such off-line workstations include core laboratory activities and smaller, single-center clinical research studies in a particular cardiology department. A schematic diagram of such a set-up is shown in Figure 10-8. A QCA workstation should be able to accept all available forms of image media.

By on-line QCA, we mean a situation in which the QCA workstation is directly connected to the image-generating X-ray system in the catheterization laboratory. This connection can be realized in different ways, from a simple analog video connection to the output of the X-ray system, which requires a selected frame to be digitized by the QCA workstation, to a preferred digital connection to the digital network of the imaging system. A schematic diagram of a networked on-line set-up is also given in Figure 10-8.

Typical applications of on-line QCA include both support of clinical decision-making during the procedure, (e.g., vessel sizing for the optimal selection of an interventional device) and an immediate assessment of the efficacy of the intervention.

FUTURE QCA DIRECTIONS

We expect extensive networking of digital review stations with and without QCA packages in the catheterization laboratory. Of course, this network will be connected to the image acquisition and viewing network of the catheterization laboratories, thereby allowing images to be transferred to the cardiologist's office and to referring hospitals. The selected images and the corresponding results can be saved on a central image server for later review and possibly reanalysis.

In terms of extension of analytical software packages, we anticipate further developments in the automated segmentation of parts of or the entire coronary tree from two (preferably orthogonal) views. This will allow the selection of optimal views for selected coronary segments and the assessment of the area of the myocardial muscle at risk. For the near future, the integration with intravascular ultrasound can be expected. On-line QCA and/or on-line quantitative intravascular ultrasound will be used increasingly to help guide the logical choice of angioplasty technology, based on lesion morphology and location in the coronary tree.

MINI COURSE

Semi-automated segmentation techniques are able to trace the luminal boundaries of coronary arteries from two-dimensional cine film or digital X-ray arteriograms after minimal user interaction.

Quantitative coronary arteriography or QCA allows the derivation of such luminal dimensions and derived indices with small systematic and random errors as demonstrated by a range of validation studies.

QCA can be used in an off-line mode for clinical research studies and in an on-line mode during the interventional procedure to support the clinical decision-making process.

SECTION FOUR

Radiation Safety

11

Radiation Biology Concepts

MICHAEL D. O'HARA[1]

INTRODUCTION

The use of ionizing radiation in the catheterization laboratory is an essential component for the diagnosis and treatment of endovascular diseases. Radiobiology is the study of how living organisms react to radiation. If ionizing radiation damages a critical cellular target such as DNA and the cell can no longer function, then cell death can occur in hours to days. If the damage to DNA results in chromosomal abnormalities, then a malignancy may be produced many years later. The purpose of this chapter is to provide the interventionalist with a review of some basic radiobiological concepts necessary to begin to understand ionizing radiation in the catheterization laboratory. The reader is encouraged to review standard textbooks for in-depth information.

RADIATION CHEMISTRY

Excitation and ionization are the two major mechanisms for energy transfer to any absorber, including living cells. Excitation refers to the elevation of electrons to a higher energy level within the atom. Electromagnetic radiation, such as ultraviolet light and visible light, transfers energy to matter in this manner. Ionizing radiation transfers sufficient energy to orbital electrons to remove them from their orbit and break chemical bonds.

There are two classes of ionizing radiation. The first is termed the particulate radiation. It includes beta particles (electrons), alpha particles (helium nuclei), neutrons, and protons. The second is termed electromagnetic radia-

[1]Research Fellow, Interventional Therapeutics, Cordis/a Johnson & Johnson Company.

tion. This class includes X-rays and gamma rays. Ionizing electromagnetic radiations have energies exceeding a few electron volts. Gamma rays originate in the nucleus of an atom and X-rays outside the atom. Except for their origin, X-rays and gamma rays are identical.

Absorption of any form of ionizing radiation (particulate or electromagnetic) in cells may result in an interaction with a biologically important target molecule. This interaction can come about two ways. The first is that the energy of the ionizing radiation can be absorbed directly by the target molecule. This is termed the direct effect. Direct ionization implies that the energy from the ionizing radiation is directly deposited into the target molecule. This effect accounts for approximately 20% of the damage done to target molecules. The indirect effect is the second way that ionizing radiation interacts with a target molecule. This effect occurs in water near the target molecule; it accounts for approximately 80% of the damage. The time frames under which these events occur are vastly different. The initial ionization step takes approximately 10^{-15} seconds. Ions have a lifetime of approximately 10^{-10} seconds and free radicals approximately 10^{-5} seconds.

The indirect effect is mediated by free radicals. A free radical is an extremely reactive, electrically neutral molecule with an unpaired electron in the outer orbital. The energy absorbed by water produces ions and free radical species that interact with the target molecule, potentially leading to biological damage of the target molecule. The breakdown of water is termed radiolysis. The end result of this interaction is the production of hydrogen (H) and hydroxyl (OH) free radicals. The free radicals can combine with each other in areas of high free radical concentration or diffuse into the nearby medium.

MOLECULAR TARGET OF RADIATION

Although a large variety of molecules or macromolecular structures can be the target of ionizing radiation, there is a great deal of evidence that DNA molecules are the primary targets.

DNA exists as a double helix of two complementary strands (i.e., twisted ladder). The supports of the ladder are composed of deoxyribose sugars and phosphate groups, whereas the rungs of the ladder are composed of nucleotides joined together by hydrogen bonds. The genetic code is contained in the sequence of the nucleotides within the rungs of the ladder. The four bases that make up the rungs of the ladder are adenine, thymine, cytocine, and guanine. Adenine bonds to thymine, and cytosine bonds to guanine.

A variety of effects of radiation on the DNA molecule have been documented. Nucleotide bases can be damaged or lost. One of the supports of the ladder can be broken, resulting in a single-strand break. Most cells can efficiently repair single-strand breaks using the complementary strand of DNA as a template. However, multiple single-strand breaks can work together to increase the amount of DNA damage. A far more serious event for an irradiated cell is when both of the strands of the ladder are broken, resulting in a double-strand break. Damaged DNA can also be cross-linked together. Damaged DNA can be visualized in many cases as chromosomal aberrations like dicentric chromosomes, acentric chromosome fragments, and ring chromosomes. Unrepaired or misrepaired DNA damage can result in the loss or alteration of genetic information.

EFFECTS ON CELL PROLIFERATION

Cell proliferation is an important component of wound healing, tissue renewal, and cancer. Tissue wounds are filled in by proliferative fibroblasts that have a limited number of replications under normal conditions. The continual renewal of circulating hematopoietic elements is under the control of bone marrow stem cells and humoral growth factors. Tumors are an example of uncontrolled proliferation limited by their ability to obtain nutrients. All three of these examples of proliferating tissues are sensitive to ionization radiation. Proliferative cells in general are sensitive to ionizing radiation. Two modes of cell death are important after exposure to ionizing radiation; these are termed reproductive death and apoptosis.

Proliferative cells exposed to massive doses of radiation die very quickly due to massive molecular damage to not only DNA but other molecular components of the cell as well. However, cells exposed to hundreds of centigrays (cGy) can.appear normal after exposure. In some cases, the cells have repaired the damage and can continue functioning normally. Other exposed cells appear normal and can continue functioning normally, even going through a few rounds of cell division. However, these cells can be damaged and incapable of continued cellular proliferation and soon die attempting a subsequent round of cell division.

The second method of cell death is termed apoptosis, also called "programmed cell death." Apoptosis is an active process that requires energy, protein, and RNA synthesis. Many external stimuli, including exposure to ionizing radiation, can induce apoptosis in a variety of normal and malignant cell types.

IN VITRO RADIOBIOLOGY

Tissue culture can be used to assess the clonogenic potential of a population of cells after exposure to ionizing radiation. A single proliferative cell placed on a tissue culture dish will eventually populate the entire surface of the dish. This can be exploited to assess the ability of a population of cells to survive an exposure to ionizing radiation. Cells growing on a tissue culture dish that survive a dose of ionizing radiation will eventually form a colony that can be identified visually. The greater the number of colonies, the higher the number of cells that survived the irradiation.

Cells from an actively growing culture can be removed from the surface of a tissue culture dish by exposure to the enzyme trypsin or other digestive enzymes to detach them from the surface of the dish. The cells are counted, and a known number of cells are inoculated onto a new tissue culture dish containing fresh medium. Multiple dishes are produced in this manner. Some of the dishes are inoculated with high numbers of cells and some with low numbers of cells. The dishes containing low numbers of cells are treated with sham radiation exposure, and, as the dose of radiation increases, the number of cells inoculated into the dishes increases. After irradiation, the cell cultures are incubated for 7–14 days. After incubation, the cultures are washed and stained. The number of colonies on each dish is determined. The plating efficiency of each dish is calculated by using the following relationship:

$$\text{Plating efficiency} = \text{colonies counted/cells seeded}$$

The plating efficiency describes the number of seeded cells that grow into colonies. The plating efficiency (PE) of each irradiated dish is compared with the plating efficiency of the control to obtain the surviving fraction using the following relationship:

$$\text{Surviving fraction} = PE_{\text{irradiated culture}}/PE_{\text{control culture}}$$

The surviving fraction can be plotted as a function of the dose in a survival curve. A representative survival curve is shown in Figure 11-1. Survival is plotted on a log scale, and dose is plotted on a linear scale. Two survival curves are plotted on Figure 11-1. *Curve H* shows the response of mammalian cells to densely ionizing (high LET) radiations like alpha particles, and *curve L* shows the survival of mammalian cells to sparsely ionizing (low LET) radiation like beta particles or gamma rays.

The survival curve for densely ionizing radiation (Fig. 11-1a, *curve H*) is an exponential function of dose. The survival curve for sparsely ionizing radiation (Fig. 11-1a, *curve L*), however, starts out as an exponential function of dose at low doses. As the dose increases, the curve starts to bend at doses exceeding a few Gy. As the dose increases further, the curve starts to straighten out again and returns to an exponential function of dose.

There are varieties of models that have been used to describe the shape of the survival curve. Most of the models can successfully predict the shape of survival curves. Biological data are not precise enough to completely fit the models. Two methods can be used to predict the shape of survival curves that have attained higher levels of acceptance. The first is termed the multitarget model, and the second is the linear-quadratic model.

The first model describes the survival curve in terms of initial slope (D_1), final slope (D_o), and the width of the shoulder (n and D_q). The initial slope (D_1) is due to a single event damaging the target, and the final slope (D_o) is due to multiple events damaging the target. These two quantities are the reciprocals of the initial and final slopes or the dose required for reduction of the surviving fraction to 37% of its original value. The extrapolation number (n) is an indicator of the width of the shoulder. The larger the value for n, the greater the width of the shoulder. The second indicator of the width of the shoulder is the quasi-threshold dose (D_q). The D_q is defined as the dose between the straight-line portion of the survival curve and the survival axis. This parameter is determined by the extrapolation of the straight-line portion of the survival curve to intersect the survival axis.

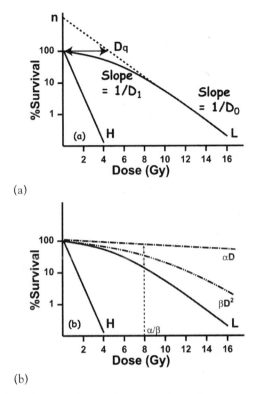

(a)

(b)

FIG. 11-1. Hypothetical survival curve for mammalian cells. Percent survival is plotted on the vertical axis and dose in Gray(Gy) on the horizontal axis. Curve H represents cell survival after irradiation with alpha particles or low energy neutrons (high LET radiation). Curve L represents cell survival after irradiation with X ray or gamma rays (low LET radiation). The descriptive parameters described by the multitarget model are shown on a and the descriptive parameters for the linear-quadratic model are shown on b.

The second model currently used to describe the shape of survival curves is called the linear-quadratic model and has gained a great deal of recent support.

This model assumes that there are two components to cell killing. The first is proportional to the dose, and the second is proportional to the square of the dose. This is directly related to chromosome aberrations in which two separate breaks are necessary to form complex aberrations. The linear-quadratic relationship defines cell survival as shown in the following equation:

$$S = e^{-\alpha D - \beta D^2}$$

where S = surviving fraction at dose D and α and β are constants.

When $\alpha D = \beta D^2$ or $D = \alpha/\beta$, the linear and quadratic contributions to cell killing are equal. The linear-quadratic model predicts a survival curve that is continuously bending.

CELL CYCLE EFFECTS

The process of cell division regulates the replication and distribution of genetic information contained within the chromosomes. As we have already seen, the DNA molecule is the most probable primary target of ionizing radiation and damage sustained by the molecule, manifest itself as chromosome aberrations, which can lead to cell death. Furthermore, duplication and segregation of the genetic material throughout the cell's life cycle both have a profound effect of the life of an irradiated cell.

The actual division of a single cell into two daughter cells (mitosis) is the only part of a cell's life cycle that is visible with a microscope. The rest of the life cycle of a cell is termed interphase. Radiolabeled DNA precursors (^{3}H-labeled thymidine) can be used to follow the fate of DNA molecules. Cultured cells are fed the radioactive thymidine. Only the cells actively synthesizing DNA will incorporate the radioactive thymidine into their DNA. The excess ^{3}H-thymidine is washed off. The cells are fixed and stained, and a thin layer of photographic emulsion is applied to coat the cells. The beta particles from the ^{3}H-thymidine enter the photographic emulsion and produce a dark "grain" above cells that have incorporated the radioactive DNA precursors. These cells, unlike cells that do not have grains above them, are the ones actively synthesizing DNA.

By incubating the cell cultures after applying the ^{3}H-thymidine, a cohort of labeled cells can be followed through their life cycle.

Another technique has replaced the ^{3}H-thymidine technique to follow the life cycle of mammalian cells. This technique uses the DNA precursor 5-bromodeoxyuridine to indicate the presence of DNA synthetic cells. A stain or an antibody to bromodeoxyuridine-substituted DNA can be applied to visualize cells that have incorporated the label.

These techniques have been used to elaborate the phases of the life cycle of mammalian cells. The cell cycle of mammalian cells is divided into four phases. These phases include the DNA synthetic phase (S phase), the phase when the mother cell separates into two daughter cells (mitosis), the gap between mitosis and the DNA synthetic phase (G_1), and the gap between the DNA synthetic phase and mitosis (G_2). Figure 11-2 shows a cartoon of a mammalian cell's life cycle. The time between successive mitoses is approxi-

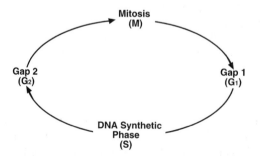

FIG. 11-2. Phases of the mitotic cycle of mammalian cells.

mately 24 hours for proliferative human cells. The lengths of each of the phases of a mammalian cell's life cycle are approximately 1, 6–8, and 4–8 hours for mitosis, S phase, and G_2, respectively. The most variable portion of a mammalian cell's life cycle is G_1, depending on the cell type and its function.

Two other cell culture techniques have been used to identify the radiation sensitivity of the phases of the life cycle of mammalian cells. These two techniques allow for the isolation of cells in a defined position within their life cycle. The first technique involves collecting mitotic cells that grow on plastic tissue culture dishes by "shaking off" the mitotic cells in a culture. This can be accomplished because many cell cultures that attach to plastic tissue culture dishes round up during mitosis and are less firmly attached to the surface of the dish. Multiple dishes can be handled in this manner to get large numbers of cells in mitosis.

Another technique that can produce large numbers of cells in the same phase of their life cycle at the same time is to use drugs. Hydroxyurea has been used for this purpose. Briefly, incubation of mammalian cells with hydroxyurea kills cells in S phase and blocks progression of surviving cells at the G_1/S boundary. Mammalian cells treated in this manner can be collected and released from the block for experimentation.

The radiation sensitivity of the various phases of the mammalian cell cycle has been determined using synchronous cells. The most resistant portion of a cell's life cycle was found to be in the last part of the S phase. Cells with a short G_1 are more sensitive to ionizing radiation than S phase cells. Cells with a longer G_1 have a second radiation-resistant period early in G_1. G_2 cells can be as sensitive as mitotic cells to ionizing radiation. The most radiation sensitive cells are cells that are irradiated in mitosis. Therefore, proliferative neointimal cells will be more sensitive to ionizing radiation than quiescent cells.

RADIATION REPAIR AND DOSE RATE EFFECTS

A large amount of irreparable radiation damage in cells is eventually lethal. However, because mammalian cells have evolved in a "sea of radiation," they have developed variable degrees of ability to repair radiation damage. There are two basic types of radiation repair. The first is called sublethal damage repair, and the second is called potentially lethal damage repair. Both of these repair mechanisms are defined by the experiment used to show their existence.

Sublethal damage repair is the repair that occurs between two doses of ionizing radiation. This type of repair can be measured using tissue culture techniques and fractionated radiation therapy. Briefly, a single dose of radiation that reduces survival to a known level is interrupted for increasing lengths of time. Instead of giving, say, 800 cGy in a single dose, 400 cGy is followed by another 400 cGy with a time interval between the two doses. Figure 11-3 is a representation of this type of experiment. *Curve A* shows a survival curve for a population of cells given a number of single doses that has a shoulder at low doses; as doses increase, the relationship between doses and survival becomes linear (exponential cell killing on a semilog plot). *Curve B* starts at 400 cGy

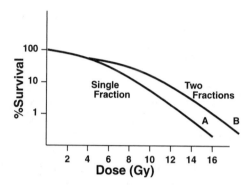

FIG. 11-3. Sublethal damage repair. Hypothetical survival data for mammalian cells: Cellular response to a single dose (A) and the same total dose delivered in two fractions (B).

given all at one time. Subsequent points on *curve B* are equivalent to the dose points on *curve A*, except fractionated into two doses separated by 2 hours. The shoulder of *curve B* is similar to *curve A*. This suggests that by providing an interval between the first half and the second half of the total dose the cells are responding to the second dose as if they have not seen the first half of the dose. If the cells could not repair the damage from the first dose, the second dose would be additive and the resulting survival would appear to fall directly on *curve A*. The terminal slope of *curve B* is identical to the terminal slope of *curve A*, but the cells have responded to the second dose of radiation as if they have never "seen" the first dose. Sublethal damage repair in mammalian cells has a half-time of approximately 1 hour in early-responding tissues and later in late-responding tissues.

Potentially lethal damage repair is also defined operationally by the experiment used to show its existence. This repair can be defined as that repair that occurs after a dose of radiation in a poor nutritional environment or in the absence of growth factors. This type of repair is most relevant to tumors or cells in the absence of growth factors. Figure 11-4 is a schematic represen-

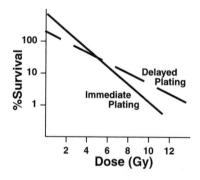

FIG. 11-4. Potentially lethal damage repair. Hypothetically; cells were irradiated in nutrient depleted medium are either immediately transferred to full growth medium (immediate plating) or left in the depleted medium for some time period before transfer to growth medium (delayed plating).

tation of an experiment. Cells were grown to confluence (stationary phase) and detached from the tissue culture dish and plated immediately after irradiation or held in stationary phase for up to 12 hours before plating. The cell cultures held for up to 12 hours in stationary phase of cell growth have a slope on the survival curve that is smaller than the slope for the cell cultures plated immediately after irradiation. This indicates that cells held in poor growth conditions (stationary phase) were able to repair the radiation damage during the time they were held in the poor growth conditions.

The rate ionizing radiation is delivered to a population of cells is one of the major determinants of how cells survive a radiation exposure. Mammalian cells are continuously irradiated by ionizing radiation delivered at extremely low dose rates from the environment and have evolved mechanisms to repair the damage. The radiation defense mechanisms of mammalian cells repair the damage with a high degree of fidelity under normal conditions, and the cells continue through their life cycles. As the dose rate increases, the ability of the cellular repair mechanisms to repair the damage is taxed and finally is exceeded. On a survival curve, as the dose rate increases, the curve gets steeper and steeper. The radiation repair mechanisms of mammalian cells acutely exposed to high dose rates (approximately 100 cGy/minute) are overwhelmed, and DNA damage goes unrepaired or is improperly repaired, resulting in division delay and cell death.

GENETIC EFFECTS OF IONIZING RADIATION

A wide variety of chemical and physical agents can produce mutations in mammalian cells. Ionizing radiation is capable of producing mutations. However, ionizing radiation does not produce new mutations that result in the production of 100-foot tall ants or grasshoppers; it increases the frequency of spontaneous mutations that already exist. The effects of radiation on the DNA molecule suggest that gene mutations or chromosomal mutations can result from radiation exposure. A gene mutation can be due to an exchange or loss of one of the bases within a DNA molecule. Changing a base or loosing a base can disrupt the sequence of amino acids in proteins that are coded for by the chain of bases within the DNA molecule, resulting in a new protein that may not perform its function or an abortive protein that cannot be used. Another type of mutation is the result of chromosomal aberrations. Chromosomal aberrations result in unusual numbers and shapes of chromosomes with the nucleus of cells.

A unique "megamouse" experiment was done at the Oak Ridge National Laboratory in the late 1950s and early 1960s with a strain of mice with seven known potential mutations that occur spontaneously. Approximately 7 million mice of both sexes were used for this study. The conclusions that can be derived from this study include the following: (1) The radiosensitivity of different mutations varies significantly from mutation to mutation; (2) there is a significant dose rate effect for mutations in the mouse; (3) prolonging the dose results in fewer mutations; and (4) males are more radiation sensitive than females, and increasing the time interval between radiation exposure and conception can reduce the genetic consequences of a dose of radiation. Furthermore, the Committee on the Biological Effects of Ionizing Radiation (BEIR V) and the United Nations Scientific Committee on the Effects of Atomic Radiation (UNSCEAR) have estimated a mutation-doubling dose of 100 cGy for low dose rate radiation.

There are few human data available to directly determine a mutation-doubling dose. The available human data suggest that the mutation doubling dose determined from animal data is approximately correct. The largest groups of humans exposed to ionizing radiation studied so far are the survivors of the atomic blasts at Hiroshima and Nagasaki. Approximately 40 years of follow-up data on the number of deaths to the age of 17, the number of untoward pregnancy outcomes, frequency of sex chromosome abnormalities, and frequency of children with blood protein electrophoretic variations have been studied in children born to survivors of the atomic blasts. The doubling doses for three of the four indicators in this population were estimated to be 800, 1500, and 2600 mSv, respectively, for untoward pregnancy outcomes, childhood mortality, and sex chromosome abnormalities.

RADIATION CARCINOGENESIS

Four possible outcomes result from exposure to ionizing radiation. The first is that the damage was fully repaired and the organism survives normally. The second is that the dose was sufficient to kill enough cells and the organism can no longer survive. The third is that the dose is not sufficient to kill a critical number of cells and the organism survives but with diminished capacity. The fourth is that the dose delivered to the organism was not fully repaired or misrepaired and a mutation has resulted. This mutation can lead to a malignancy.

Survival with diminished capacity is an example of a deterministic effect of radiation. The deterministic effects have a threshold dose below which there is no probability of observable harm. Above the threshold dose, increasing the dose further increases the probability and severity of the effect. The mutation that leads to a malignancy is an example of a stochastic effect. Stochastic effects such as production of malignancies (carcinogenesis) and mutation (hereditary changes) increase in frequency with dose but do not increase in severity as a function of dose. Within a few years of the discovery of X-rays by Roentgen, varieties of deterministic and stochastic effects were observed. Some of the early deterministic effects observed include dermatitis, epilation, and anemia. Skin cancer and leukemia are examples of some of the first stochastic effects of radiation exposure observed.

There is a well-known and poorly understood link between cancer and radiation exposure. Much of our understanding about the link between cancer and radiation exposure comes from accidental exposure to early radiation workers, medical accidents, and exposure as a result of the atomic bomb blasts at Hiroshima and Nagasaki. A variety of cancers have been linked to radiation exposure of humans.

The first human cancer to be linked to radiation exposure was skin cancer. Early radiation workers suffered chronic radiodermatitis, which, after a long latent period, resulted in squamous cell and basal cell carcinoma. Skin cancers are readily accessible and can be diagnosed and treated at an early stage. However, significant improvement in radiation safety has resulted in very little skin cancer in radiation workers today. Survivors of the atomic blasts at Hiroshima and Nagasaki have not shown increased susceptibility to skin cancers as a result of their exposure.

The thyroid gland is amongst the most radiation sensitive tissue in terms of radiation-induced cancer. Radiation-induced thyroid tumors develop slowly and are well differentiated. These tumors can be successfully treated with surgery or radioactive iodine. A number of different exposed groups have contributed to our understanding of radiation-induced thyroid cancer. These groups include survivors of the atomic blasts at Hiroshima and Nagasaki, the Marshall Islanders exposed to radioactive iodine fallout from thermonuclear device testing, the children exposed to X-rays to treat an enlarged thymus, and the children treated with X-rays for enlarged tonsils and nasopharynx or the children treated with X-rays for tinea capitis.

Another tissue that may be very sensitive to radiation-induced cancer formation is the breast. Three populations of humans have contributed to our understanding of the relationship between radiation exposure and breast cancer. The first are the female patients exposed to multiple fluoroscopies for diagnosis and treatment of pulmonary tuberculosis in Nova Scotia and Massachusetts. Many of these women received approximately 100 fluoroscopies and some received over 500 fluoroscopies. The second group of women exposed to radiation were those exposed as a result of the atomic blasts at Hiroshima and Nagasaki. The last group of women to show an increase in breast cancer as a result of radiation exposure were those exposed to ionizing radiation for the treatment of postpartum mastitis.

Many agents have been linked to lung cancer, and radiation is one of them. Three groups of humans exposed to radiation have contributed to our understanding of the risk of radiation-induced lung cancer. The first are the survivors of the atomic blasts at Hiroshima and Nagasaki. The second are patients treated with ionizing radiation for ankylosing spondylysis, and the third are miners who were exposed to high concentrations of radon gas in uranium mines. The risk assessment from the uranium miners has also been used to justify radon reduction systems in private homes. However, the miners were exposed to far greater concentrations of radon gas and other known carcinogens.

Bone cancer has also been linked to radiation exposure. The exposed populations that have contributed to our understanding of the risk of bone cancer after exposure to ionizing are the young women that were employed as radium watch dial painters and the patients treated with radium-224 for the treatment of tuberculosis or ankylosing spondylysis. The radium watch dial painters dipped their brushes into paints containing radium to put luminous dials on watches. To make well-defined luminescent dots, the painters would lick the brushes to get a sharp point. This group was found to have a much higher number of bone tumors compared with the general public.

Leukemia has also been shown to be a result of radiation exposure. Leukemia has the shortest latent period of any of the radiation-induced tumors, approximately 7–12 years. Two groups demonstrate that some types of leukemia can be the result of radiation exposure. The first are the atomic blast survivors at Hiroshima and Nagasaki, and the second are patients that were treated for ankylosing spondylysis. Acute and chronic myeloid leukemia are the most prevalent types of leukemia linked to adult human radiation exposure. Acute lymphocytic leukemia is the most prevalent leukemia linked to childhood exposure to radiation, and chronic lymphocytic leukemia does not appear to be linked to radiation exposure.

The risk of radiation-induced tumors resulting from radiation exposure has been estimated by the United Nations Scientific Committee on the Effects of Atomic Radiations (UNSCEAR) and the Committee on the Biological Effects of Ionizing Radiation (BEIR). The lifetime risk of fatality from cancer varies with both dose rate and the age distribution of the irradiated population. The per-sievert estimates of risk range from 5×10^{-2} to 10×10^{-2}. To scale this risk, a radiation worker receiving the entire International Commission on Radiation Protection (ICRP) maximum permissible dose of 0.01 Sv per year for 40 years has an estimated 3% radiogenic cancer risk. In comparison, the "natural" cancer risk is approximately 30%.

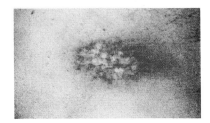

FIG. 12-1. **Poikilodermic lesion below the right axilla (7.5 × 3.5 cm).** 5–6 years after two PTCA procedures. With permission from *Arch Dermatol* 132;663–667. Copyrighted 1996, American Medical Association.

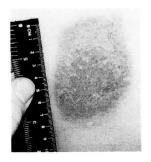
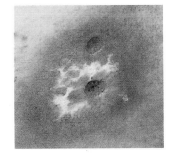

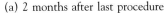

(a) 2 months after last procedure   (b) 5 months

FIG. 12-2. **Diabetic patient who developed stenoses in her coronary vessels and venous bypass grafts.** Angioplasties and coronary stent placements were performed in two sessions separated by 1 month [Stone MS et al.].

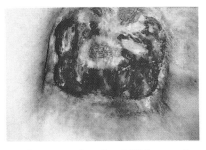

FIG. 12-3. **Radiation wound 13 months after TIPS procedure.** Corpulent patient with multiple health problems [Wagner LK et al.].

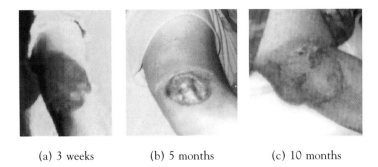

(a) 3 weeks   (b) 5 months   (c) 10 months

FIG. 12-4. Arm of a patient who underwent electrophysiological ablation treatment for cardiac arrhythmia. Arm was in direct beam near x-ray port. a: 3 weeks after procedure. b: 5 months later dermal necrosis is evident. c: Skin flap at 10 months [Wagner LK et al.].

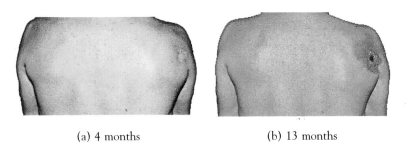

(a) 4 months   (b) 13 months

FIG. 12-5. PTCA Injury after treatment of the left circumflex artery. [Wolff D, et al.] a: 4 months; b: 13 months.

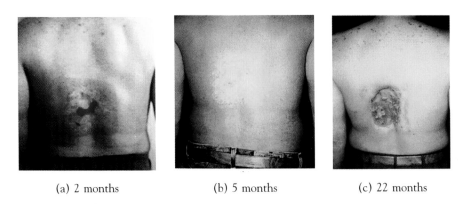

(a) 2 months   (b) 5 months   (c) 22 months

FIG. 12-6. Post angioplasty. [Shope TB] a: 2 months; b: five months; c: 22 months.

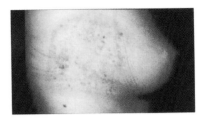

FIG. 12-7. Fluoroscopically guided electrophysiological ablation. Seventeen-year-old woman 2 years after unsuccessful attempts to treat her cardiac arrhythmia. The patient had difficulty raising her right arm [Vañó E et al.].

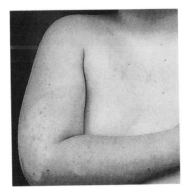

FIG. 12-8. Arm of 7-year-old girl who underwent cadiological ablation procedure with beam positioned laterally, passing through her arm [Vañó E et al.].

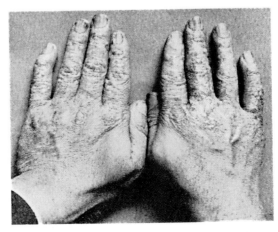

FIG. 12-9. Hands of Mirhan Krikor Kassabian. Age 33 years and about 7 years after starting work with fluoroscopy [Kassabian MK].

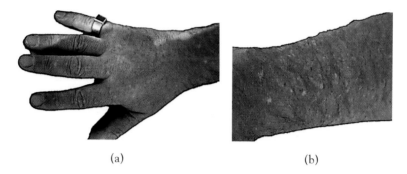

(a)   (b)

FIG. 12-10. Hand and arm of a pain management interventionalist. This individual has been in practice for more than 20 years (digitally enhanced to demonstrate radiation induced changes) [Photo supplied by Balter].

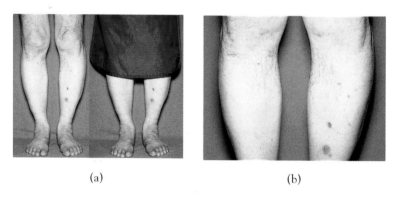

(a)   (b)

FIG. 12-11. Legs of an interventionalist after 40 years of practice. Note the distinct line of hair loss below the lead apron [Photo supplied by subject].

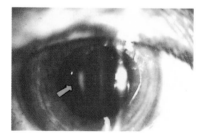

FIG. 12-12. Radiation-induced cataract in an interventional fluoroscopist (arrow) [Vañó E et al.].

12

Radiation Injuries From Fluoroscopy: A 21st Century Déjà Vu

LOUIS K. WAGNER[1] and TITUS R. KOENIG[1]

INTRODUCTION

Since about 1990, the burgeoning expansion of fluoroscopically guided interventional procedures has been accompanied by numerous incidences of radiation-induced injuries in patients and in medical personnel. The types of injuries range from mild skin changes, such as epilation, to serious debilitating injuries, such as deep dermal necroses that require musculocutaneous skin grafting after a prolonged period of nonhealing skin ulceration. In one case even resection of a rib was necessary in order to achieve healing. In almost all of these cases, physicians did not initially recognize the injury as related to radiation. In fact, many physicians are of the belief that fluoroscopy is such a "low-dose" procedure that such effects are impossible with today's technology. The evidence clearly speaks otherwise.

Fluoroscopic injury is a well-documented phenomenon that became apparent very shortly after Roentgen discovered the X ray in 1895. With time, physicians and researchers learned how to better design equipment and to protect themselves against radiation. As the use of X rays expanded, more challenges on protection of the patient and the physician developed. In the 1960s, reports of radiation-induced breast cancer from interventional use of fluoroscopy surfaced, pointing to the continued need for increasing benefit by reducing risks. In the 1960s, government regulations on the design performance of fluoroscopic units defined standards that helped reduce the likelihood of

[1]University of Texas, Houston, TX
This chapter is dedicated to Dr. Kassabian and his message of prevention.

injury from the use of this equipment. The application of fluoroscopy was mostly for diagnostic work for which the duration of fluoroscopic exposure was relatively brief. From about 1960 through 1990, the frequency of reported injuries in patients and personnel was so low that the success in reducing risk led many to a false sense of security that the problem was solved. However, medical practice changed in the 1980s with the introduction of many new fluoroscopically guided interventional techniques. These required much longer use of the fluoroscope than previously required for conventional diagnostic purposes. With sophisticated minimally invasive medical devices, high-technology, high-capacity X-ray tubes, and the introduction of immediate-acquisition-and-review digital imaging techniques, the stage was set for a recurrence of events common during the late 1890s and early 20th century.

This chapter reviews the types of injuries that have been caused by fluoroscopy so that medical staff can recognize these injuries and take follow-up actions to reduce the frequency and severity of occurrence.

DETERMINISTIC EFFECTS

Radiation injury from fluoroscopy is called a deterministic effect. Examples of deterministic effects include erythema, cataract, epilation, telangiectasia, ulcers, and necrosis. Deterministic effects are characterized by the following:

- They do not occur unless the amount of radiation exceeds a certain level, referred to as a threshold. This is because their occurrence requires that many cells be severely injured before the effect can manifest itself. They do not occur when the dose of radiation is below the threshold for the effect. Different thresholds apply to different effects.
- The probability of observing the effect increases as the radiation dose increases beyond the threshold. As dose increases, more cells are injured, increasing the likelihood of the event.
- If the dose is sufficient to cause an effect, the severity of the effect increases as dose continues to increase.
- When the dose is sufficiently beyond the threshold, the effect will be seen in 100% of exposed individuals.

The two organs of principal concern for deterministic effects are skin and lens of the eye. The reason for this is that the X-ray beams used in fluoroscopy deposit most of their energy in the surface layers of tissue where the beam enters the body, rendering the skin and eyes most likely to receive a high dose. In addition, effects are easily noticed in these external organs, even though they may not necessarily cause any sensations in the affected individual.

Other organs of concern for late effects, especially when under 20 years of age at time of irradiation, include the breast (female), bone marrow, thyroid, brain, and growing bone. Radiation-induced cancer, not a deterministic effect, is the primary concern and the potential for bone growth retardation in children may be a sequela if doses to growing bone are sufficiently high. For example, children undergoing interventional procedures in the head may be at risk. When doses are very high, the lung and spine may be at risk. Severe skin effects would precede effects in these organs. Parotid glands may also show effects, resulting in dry mouth and swelling.

Recognizing mild forms of radiation-induced skin injury can be useful in the management of patients and in the modification of radiation protection habits of personnel. For example, patients who undergo multiple interventions may demonstrate skin changes from initial procedures that render the skin at risk for more serious injury from additional interventions. Actions might be taken to prevent irradiation of the affected site. If personnel demonstrate radiation-induced changes in themselves, recognition of these changes will force action to improve radiation safety practices. Examples of these situations will be demonstrated later.

MECHANISM OF RADIATION ENERGY DEPOSITION

While radiation is applied, patients or personnel have no sensation that a radiation injury is being induced. This runs counterintuitive to our experiences with heat. On an elementary scale, one might be led to believe that the mechanisms for thermal burns are the same as those for fluoroscopy-induced radiation "burns." They are not the same at all. The deposition of heat from a flame causes an external rise in temperature that superficial nerves can sense to provide a safety alarm to an exposed individual. Fluoroscopic radiation does not cause this temperature rise. For example, a threshold dose of about 6 gray (Gy) to the epidermis is required to induce an erythema that results from basal cell depletion. This dose will raise the temperature of the exposed epidermal skin area by a mere 0.002°C.

How, then, can such a small deposition of energy cause such a dramatic biological change? The answer lies in the mechanism of injury. Heat has to work its way into a cell from the outside. X rays do not do this. X rays deposit their energy at the biomolecular level. This interaction is sufficient to break molecular bonds and cause changes in the biochemistry of the cell without raising its temperature. These biochemical changes, when sufficiently extensive, can cause cell dysfunction and cell death.

UNDERSTANDING FLUOROSCOPIC INJURIES

Dependence on Dose, Dose Rate and Tissue Type

The concept that the degree of injury is related to the dose of radiation is intuitive. However, factors such as dose rate, dose fractionation, and tissue sensitivity play essential roles in the outcome of a radiation exposure. This stems from the ability of a cell to recover from an ionizing event and other cellular repair mechanisms, such as replacement of damaged cells. If the radiation dose rate is sufficiently low, cellular repair mechanisms can manage the ionization insult more effectively than when the rate of ionization is more intense. Thus, the same dose delivered at a high rate will cause a more severe effect than when delivered at a low dose rate. This also means that the cumulated dose threshold for inducing the effect will be greater for lower dose rates. A similar situation occurs for fractionation of a dose. When a dose is delivered in two or more separate sessions separated by many days, tissue healing plays an important role in preparing the affected tissue for further irradiation. Thus, a very high dose of fluoroscopic X rays delivered in a single procedure will produce a more severe response than that same dose delivered in three separate sessions separated by months.

For medical personnel, the dose is usually delivered at low dose rates fractionated daily. The thresholds for effects will therefore be higher than those anticipated from acute delivery. Despite these facts, cataracts and severe radiation-induced effects in hands have been observed relatively recently in medical personnel. Effects in the legs and feet of personnel have also been observed.

The sensitivity of tissues to X rays varies with the tissue type and with the characteristics of the individual. Age, disease, and medication all can play a role. The young have greater reserves of healthy tissue and recover more efficiently from an injury. Skin on the back of the hand is more sensitive than that on the palm. Patients with collagen vascular disease, diabetes mellitus, and patients homozygous for ataxia telangiectasia are at heightened risk for adverse reactions to X rays.

Delay From Irradiation to Appearance of Injury

The appearance of a radiation-induced injury is usually delayed with respect to the time of irradiation. This delay is related to the biological mechanisms and temporal patterns of cell function, replication, degeneration, and repair. Because different tissues in the skin differ with respect to all these aspects, the time course of the development of the injury can be a series of changes as different tissues respond to the radiation damage. Of course, the promptness and the severity of the changes will depend on dose and dose rate.

SKIN INJURIES

A summary of skin injuries is given in Table 12-1.

Early Erythema—Threshold of ~2 Gy

The first response of skin to a mildly high level of an acute fluoroscopic dose in the range of 2 Gy is an activation of histamine-like substances, resulting in permeability and dilation of small vessels. This manifests itself as a transient erythema that is well known in radiation therapy. This type of response may begin promptly after irradiation, within hours, and usually peaks at about 24 h, after which it may quickly recede. As always, the time course and severity depend on dose and dose rate. At doses near the threshold, it may appear only

TABLE 12-1. Threshold skin entrance doses for different skin injuries

Effect	Single-dose Threshold (Gy)	Onset
Early transient erythema	2	2–24 hours
Main Erythema	6	~10 d
Temporary epilation	3	~3 wk
Permanent epilation	7	~3 wk
Dry desquamation	14	~4 wk
Moist desquamation	18	~4 wk
Secondary ulceration	24	>6 wk
Late erythema	15	8–10 wk
Ischemic dermal necrosis	18	>10 wk
Dermal atrophy (1st phase)	10	>12 wk
Dermal atrophy (2nd phase)	10	>1 yr
Induration (Invasive Fibrosis)	10	
Telangiectasia	10	>1 yr
Late dermal necrosis	>12?	>1 yr
Skin cancer	not known	>5 yr

(Adapted from Wagner LK, Eifel PJ, Geise RA. Potential biological effects following high x-ray dose interventional procedures. JVIR 1994; 5:71–84 with updated revisions based on private communication with John Hopewell.)

as a blush. At very high doses, it may blend with the main erythematous effect that is a reaction due to depletion of basal cells in the epidermis. Some interventionalists have described effects that appear to be this type of response, but we know of no confirmation of this effect for fluoroscopically guided interventional work. This may be due to its transient nature.

Epilation—Threshold of ~3 Gy

As dose increases to the acute threshold of about 3 Gy, hair depletion begins. Radiation-induced recoverable hair loss in the dean at Vanderbilt University in 1896 was one of the very first documented radiation-induced effects. The sensitive cells are in the germinal layer of the hair follicle. When replicative function of these cells is destroyed by X rays, the number of cells available for hair growth is diminished and the hair at the follicle is thinner. When sufficiently deprived of cells, the hair is weak and tends to break off at the skin line, resulting in hair loss. The evolution of this effect follows the course of hair growth, and the onset of the effect occurs at about 3 weeks. Recovery is apparent at about 6 weeks. As dose increases, cell depletion increases and recovery may not be complete, resulting in permanently thinner hair. At about 7 Gy, total elimination of the germinal layer is possible, with no recovery and permanent loss of hair in the affected follicle.

Hair loss is more of a cosmetic consequence than a serious health threat. It has been observed in patients undergoing interventional procedures in the head and on the back of some who have undergone cardiological interventions. The sensitivity of hair is related to growth rate, with faster-growing hair being more sensitive. Hair follicles of the scalp appear to be of higher sensitivity than other hair.

Erythema—The Main Effect With Threshold of ~6 Gy

As acute dose delivery increases to a threshold of about 6 Gy, a delayed erythema may occur and begins within about 10 days. This erythema is believed to be in response to depletion of the basal cells of the epidermis. The inflammatory response is the skin's mechanism for hastening repopulation of the cells.

Desquamation—Threshold of ~14 Gy

As dose increases, more basal cells are affected. This seriously limits the skin's ability to regenerate, and a dry desquamation may occur at threshold doses of about 14 Gy. At greater doses, the damage becomes sufficiently extensive to result in vesicles and a moist desquamation (~18 Gy). Onset occurs at around 4 weeks.

Secondary Ulceration—Threshold of ~24 Gy

When skin is sufficiently injured, the overlying epidermis is weak, skin sloughing occurs, and the tissue is susceptible to minor injury. There is an increased risk for infection. This may result in ulceration that becomes apparent at around 6 weeks or later after irradiation. Ulcers may heal and recur several times over a period of months to years, often following light trauma or exposure to ultraviolet light.

Late Erythema—Threshold of ~15 Gy

If dose is about 15 Gy or greater, a third phase of erythema may develop 8–10 weeks after irradiation. It is associated with a dusky or mauve discoloration due to edema.

Ischemic Dermal Necrosis—Threshold of ~18 Gy

Beginning about 10–16 weeks after irradiation to doses in excess of 18 Gy, there may be an increasing loss of endothelial cells and reduction in the capillary density. Proliferating viable endothelial cells occlude the endarterioles. This vascular insufficiency leads to dermal ischemia and necrosis.

Dermal Atrophy—Threshold of ~10 Gy

Doses that do not result in ulceration may still result in dermal atrophy. This is particularly likely if moist desquamation occurs. It may occur as early as 3 months after irradiation or may gradually progress for years. This effect may have two phases. The epidermis is reduced to a few cell layers void of hair. Focal deposition of melanin may give the skin a discolored (poikilodermic) appearance.

Induration (Invasive Fibrosis)—Threshold of ~10 Gy

Dermal and subcutaneous induration is a healing response seen after ulceration and dermal necrosis, although milder forms are apparent after doses of about 10 Gy. It commonly progresses with time. The skin and subcutaneous fat feels woodlike on palpation. The area is acutely tender. It can lead to a marked decrease in the range of movement if it occurs close to joints.

Telangiectasia—Threshold of ~10 Gy

Skin telangiectasia is induced at doses of about 10 Gy. It has been reported to occur as early as about 4 months after interventional procedures in some patients, but it usually becomes visible after about 1 year, often increasing in extent as time progresses. This progression may last for more than 10 years.

Late Dermal Necrosis—Threshold of ~12 Gy

Even if doses are insufficient to result in desquamation, ulceration, or necrosis in the first 12 months, a late phase of dermal necrosis may still occur. The threshold for this effect is less well investigated than other thresholds. The best estimate at this time is about 12 Gy.

Sensitive Patients

The likelihood of skin injury, particularly severe injury, is greater in patients with certain diseases. Two potential mechanisms for this susceptibility may be greater genetic susceptibility to injury and a compromised healing process. Some of the diseases of greatest concern are collagen vascular disease (connective tissue diseases such as lupus erythematosus, scleroderma, mixed connective tissue disease, and possibly rheumatoid arthritis), diabetes mellitus, and the homozygous form of ataxia telangiectasia. In one such case, a gentleman developed dermal necrosis and required rib resection after a transjugular portosystemic shunt placement that employed a high radiation dose. However, the dose was thought to have been too low to cause that type of injury in normal skin. The wound remained open for about 4 years before it was successfully covered with a skin transplant.

Sensitivities of Different Skin Tissues

Radiation sensitivity varies among different sites on the body. The most radiosensitive areas are anterior neck, antecubital and popliteal areas, and the flexor surfaces of the extremities. Next in radiosensitivity is the chest and abdomen, followed by the face, then the back and the extensor surfaces of the extremities, and then the nape of the neck and the scalp. Finally, the palms and soles are least sensitive. Scalp hair is more radiosensitive than hair on other parts of the body.

Serious radiation injuries to patients are most frequently reported for cardiac procedures and transjugular intrahepatic portosystemic shunt (TIPS) placements. For these procedures, the skin areas receiving the highest doses are the back and axillae, which are more radiosensitive than the scalp, except for hair loss. Epilation has been observed periodically in patients undergoing neurointerventional procedures, but the only serious injury reported for neurointerventional work occurred in the lumbar spine area, where the skin is more sensitive. We know of no serious injuries in the scalp. These observations are likely to be a reflection of several important factors, including differences in the radiosensitivity of the different irradiated skin areas, differences in body habitus, with the thicker abdominal and thoracic parts requiring higher dose rates to penetrate the anatomy, as well as several other important differences related to radiation delivery.

SKIN CANCER—A STOCHASTIC EFFECT

Radiation-induced skin cancer is believed to be a stochastic effect, not a deterministic effect. That is, within the limitations of our knowledge, it is theoretically possible that any dose of X rays could induce skin cancer. Basal and squamous cell carcinomas are known to be induced; melanoma has not been identified as an x-ray radiation-induced cancer. Induction at low doses is extremely unlikely. If skin injury does occur, the likelihood for developing cancer is markedly increased and becomes a greater concern.

CATARACT

In this chapter, a cataract is any opacity of the lens of the eye that can be detected under a slit-lamp microscope. A cataract may or may not be vision impairing.

The human lens is an ovoid-shaped organ at the center of which is a nucleus surrounded by layering cells. This layering takes on the style of an onion. While production of cells in the lens may occur throughout life, removal of cells is not known to occur. Cells injured by radiation lose their lucency and migrate to the posterior pole where the cataract is observed to begin. Doses in excess of 1 Gy, delivered acutely, are necessary to produce a minimal cataract in an otherwise healthy lens. The threshold for induction is greater when irradiation is administered in low-dose rates over extended periods. Latency and progression are also expected to be affected by dose rate. The progression of cataracts depends on dose level. A small percentage (~10%) become progressive for doses between 2 and 5 Gy. Stationary (nonprogressing) cataracts may result in little to no vision impairment. The time between irradiation and diagnosis is at least 6 months, but the average time is about 8 years for doses less than about 6 Gy. The average latent period is shorter as dose increases.

CASE REPORTS

With the burgeoning growth of interventional fluoroscopy, there has been a resurgence in radiation injuries to patients and physicians. Within the published peer-reviewed journals and through other means, such as other academic research and lawsuits, at least 70 cases of radiation injury to patients were known at the time of this publication. Many radiation effects in medical personnel have also been reported. These range from mild changes in the skin, such as hair loss and color changes in the legs, to cataracts and severe skin injuries in the hands. Some of these cases are summarized below to illustrate the types of skin changes possible.

Patients

Case 1

Lichtenstein and others reported on a patient who had a 7.5 × 3.5-cm skin lesion of a poikilodermic nature located below the right axilla. The patient noticed the lesion 1.5 years after the second of two percutaneous transluminal coronary angioplasties (PTCA) procedures (Fig. 12-1). The procedures occurred a year apart from each other. The patient had not associated the lesion with the cardiac procedures, and it remained asymptomatic for 5–6 years before the patient sought medical attention for pain. At the time of examination, epidermal atrophy, telangiectasia, and dyspigmentation were noted. Histological findings were also consistent with a diagnosis of chronic radiation injury.

This case illustrates that asymptomatic changes occur and can result in symptoms years after procedures are completed. They can progress over extended periods of time into painful lesions. This type of injury can only be avoided if skin dose is kept below thresholds for this type of change (~10 Gy). Recognition of such lesions will help in prevention of more serious skin injury if future procedures can avoid irradiation of the same site.

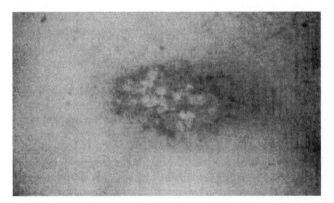

FIG. 12-1. Poikilodermic lesion below the right axilla (7.5 × 3.5 cm). 5–6 years after two PTCA procedures. With permission from *Arch Dermatol* 132;663–667. Copyrighted 1996, American Medical Association. Figure also appears in Color Figure section.

Case 2

Stone et al described a radiation-induced injury in a diabetic patient who developed chest pain as a result of stenoses in her coronary vessels and her

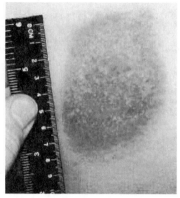 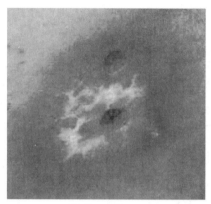

(a) 2 months after last procedure   (b) 5 months

FIG. 12-2. Diabetic patient who developed stenoses in her coronary vessels and venous bypass grafts. Angioplasties and coronary stent placements were performed in two sessions separated by 1 month [Stone MS et al.]. Figures also appear in Color Figure section.

bypass grafts of a previous surgery. Angioplasties and coronary stent placements were performed in two sessions separated by 1 month. About 1 week after her last procedure, she observed an erythematous area on the left side of her back. This persisted and was painful. At 2 months (Fig. 12-2a), desquamation was evident. By 7 months, the borders of the lesion measured 7 × 7 cm and were hyperpigmented. The central area was warm and very tender with areas of erythema, dyspigmentation, and telangiectasia. Two shallow 1-cm-ulcers were present which enlarged over the subsequent course. (Fig. 12-2b). Dose to the skin was estimated to be in the range of 10 Gy.

Notable in this case is that the patient had diabetes, which has been identified in radiation therapy as a potentiator for radiation-related complications. Also notable is that multiple stenting and angioplasty procedures were involved. These factors place the patient at elevated risk for injury. The temporal patterns observed in this case are similar to those seen in other cases.

Case 3

Wagner and coauthors discussed a corpulent patient with multiple health problems who later developed a highly unusual reaction to radiation. The patient's health status included diabetes mellitus, mixed connective tissue disease, Sjogren syndrome, hepatic cirrhosis of nonalcoholic origin, and portal hypertension.

During a second hospitalization for his esophageal varices, the patient underwent superior mesenteric angiography, hepatic venography, and liver biopsy. Three weeks later, the patient reported to a dermatologist's office with an intensely pruritic area on his back, which was diagnosed as contact dermatitis but which is now known to have been related to his earlier angiographic procedure. Six months later, the patient had a recurrent episode of hematemesis and underwent a TIPS procedure. The procedure proved to be difficult, lasting 5 hours. On the following day, the patient had developed a warm

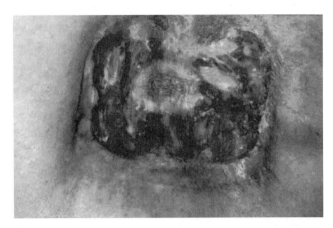

FIG. 12-3. Radiation wound 13 months after TIPS procedure. Corpulent patient with multiple health problems [Wagner LK et al.]. Figure also appears in Color Figure section.

pruritic erythematous area about 10 × 15 cm on his back where the X-ray beam had entered. The rash persisted and developed into a deep necrotic wound over a protracted time course of 5 years. The wound exposed ribs, at least one of which was subsequently resected (Fig. 12-3). Radiation dose analysis did not reveal any condition likely to have led to a radiation level that would be sufficient to cause such an event in healthy skin.

This patient was not a good candidate for conventional surgery due to his multiple health problems. Some of these conditions are believed to be responsible for sensitizing the patient to radiation and thus leading to the unusual reaction (see previous discussion). Screening patients for a history of diseases as specified earlier may help identify some patients who may be at added risk for radiation complications in long procedures. At a minimum, such information should be used in counseling patients before fluoroscopically guided interventional work.

Case 4

Wagner and Archer described an injury to the arm of a patient who underwent a treatment for cardiac arrhythmia. The patient was restless despite conscious sedation. Her hands were initially supported over her abdomen with arms resting in this position. After the sterile drapes were positioned, her restlessness apparently caused her right arm to relax off the side of the table. The elbow came to rest on the port of the X-ray tube that had its separator cone removed. This placed the elbow within about 20–25 cm of the source. Only about 20 minutes of fluoroscopy from this projection were used for the procedure, which lasted 6 hours.

In this position, the intensity of the X-ray source was very high because of the added absorption of the arm, which drove the output to or near its maximum, and because of the close proximity of the skin to the source. The patient was released the following day after a successful treatment. The patient had no complaints at the time of release.

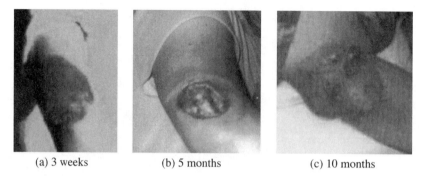

(a) 3 weeks   (b) 5 months   (c) 10 months

FIG. 12-4. Arm of a patient who underwent electrophysiological ablation treatment for cardiac arrhythmia. Arm was in direct beam near x-ray port. a: 3 weeks after procedure. b: 5 months later dermal necrosis is evident. c: Skin flap at 10 months [Wagner LK et al.]. Figures also appear in Color Figure section.

Three weeks later, an intense erythema was present above her right elbow (Fig. 12-4a). Five months later, dermal necrosis was evident (Fig. 12-4b). Figure 12-4c shows the surgical skin flap at 10 months.

The surprising factor of this injury is that no one in the room during the procedure was aware that the arm was in the direct beam. This could have been due to the fact that the humerus was very magnified on the video monitor and no one recognized the bone for what it was. On some magnification levels, the magnified bone could cover the displayed image field.

This episode dramatically demonstrates the need for physicians and ancillary personnel to be trained in the recognition of extraneous anatomy under all magnified conditions and to realize that circumstances like this can cause unnecessary, and even dangerous, levels of irradiation. It also points out the need to understand the purpose of the separator cone and the precautions that must be observed if it is removed.

Case 5

Wolff and Heinrich described a patient who underwent PTCA to treat a stenosis of the left circumflex artery. The fluoroscopy time was recorded at 51 minutes. With the X-ray c-arm in the left anterior oblique orientation, the beam entered the back at the right shoulder. Fourteen days later, an erythema developed that worsened with time. By 4 months, (Fig. 12-5a), the area demonstrated a depressed atrophied plaque surrounded by hyperpigmentation. The lesion progressed into an area of deep dermal necrosis (Fig. 12-5b).

Several injuries of this type have appeared in the literature. High-dose rates occur in these patients because the shoulder is close to the X-ray port and the density and amount of tissue that must be penetrated is large with these types of beam orientations. Exposure rates can be very high. Prolonged irradiation of the same skin area should be avoided. If possible, the beam should be rotated slightly to prevent overirradiation of any one area. Real-time dose monitoring would be a great help in warning physicians about the radiation doses during such cases. This would at least give the physician the

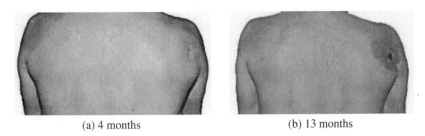

(a) 4 months   (b) 13 months

FIG. 12-5. PTCA **Injury after treatment of the left circumflex artery.** [Wolff D, et al.] a: 4 months; b: 13 months. Figures also appear in Color Figure section.

option of knowing when to change the orientation to avoid further irradiation of heavily dosed areas.

Case 6

Shope reported on a 75-kg patient who underwent three angioplasty treatments and subsequently developed a large area of deep skin necrosis. About 5 months after the first balloon angioplasty of the right coronary artery, the patient was admitted for balloon angioplasty of the left anterior descending artery. Shortly after completion of the second procedure, the patient developed chest pain and a third angioplasty procedure was started. This was unsuccessful, and the patient was sent to surgery for emergency bypass. At the time of transfer, the medical staff noted an erythema on the patient's back. The cumulated fluoroscopy time was about 1 hour. This initial erythema apparently faded because the area was described later as having turned red at about 1 month and peeling 1 week later. At 2 months, the area had the appearance of a second-degree burn (Fig. 12-6a). The wound then seemed to recover somewhat, demonstrating atrophic dyspigmented epidermal healing with a central area of ulceration (Fig. 12-6b). As time progressed, dermal necrosis developed (Fig. 12–6c). The wound was covered successfully with a skin graft about 2 years after the last angioplasty procedure.

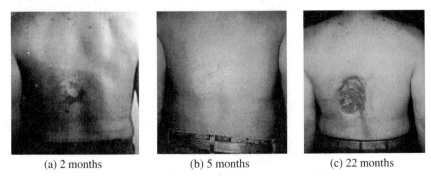

(a) 2 months   (b) 5 months   (c) 22 months

FIG. 12-6. Post angioplasty. [Shope TB] a: 2 months; b: five months; c: 22 months. Figures also appear in Color Figure section.

A retrospective dose assessment was not possible due to a lack of information about the status of the equipment at the time of the procedure, which may have included high-dose-rate fluoroscopy.

Knowledge about how dose and dose rate relate to the equipment and positioning of the patient relative to the X-ray beam is essential to properly manage radiation delivery. Almost all modern fluoroscopes have multiple dose-rate settings to control dose rate and image quality. Physicians who operate fluoroscopes must have machine-specific knowledge of these features in order to manage radiation delivery properly.

Case 7

Vañó and coauthors discussed the case of a 17-year-old woman who underwent two unsuccessful attempts to treat her cardiac arrhythmia with fluoroscopically guided electrophysiological ablation. The fluoroscopy time summed to about 100 minutes, and the entrance skin dose was estimated at 11–15 Gy. About 12 hours after the second attempt, an erythema developed in the area of the right axilla. At 4 weeks, the area was red and blistering. After 2 years, a 5-cm × 10-cm poikilodermic, atrophic, indurated plaque remained (Fig. 12-7). The patient had difficulty raising her right arm.

This is a very important example of the persistent nature of such injuries and the complex risks involved. The axilla is one of the more radiation sensitive areas of the body, and the poor healing resulted in impairment of arm movement. Furthermore, the female breast is one of the more radiosensitive organs for radiation-induced cancer, and women and girls under the age of 20 are the most sensitive age group. In the first half of the 20th century, radiation-induced breast cancer was caused by fluoroscopy in women treated for pulmonary tuberculosis using fluoroscopically guided artificial pneumothorax. After about age 25, this patient will be at elevated risk for developing breast cancer. This risk appears to persist for many decades.

Sometimes during interventional procedures in the thorax, the female breast is directly in the X-ray beam. Moreover, sometimes the breast is in the intense entrance beam. A conscientious effort to avoid direct irradiation, es-

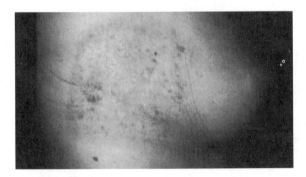

FIG. 12-7. Fluoroscopically guided electrophysiological ablation. Seventeen-year-old woman 2 years after unsuccessful attempts to treat her cardiac arrhythmia. The patient had difficulty raising her right arm [Vañó E et al.]. Figure also appears in Color Figure section.

pecially entrance beam irradiation, would well serve the health interests of the patient.

Case 8

Vañó and coauthors also discussed the circumstances of a 7-year-old girl who had a cardiac ablation procedure. The procedure was performed with the X-ray tube laterally projecting through her right arm. The fluoroscopy on-time was 75–100 minutes. Four months later, the patient returned with an indurated erythematous plaque on her right arm where the beam entered (Fig. 12-8).

This is a second case of a patient whose arm was in the direct beam near the port during the procedure. The added tissue and the proximity of the arm to the port both combine to seriously increase dose rate to the skin. Moving arms out of the way of the beam can be a difficult task. A concerted effort to accommodate a comfortable support for the arm without compromising circulation is an essential task to avoid such injuries.

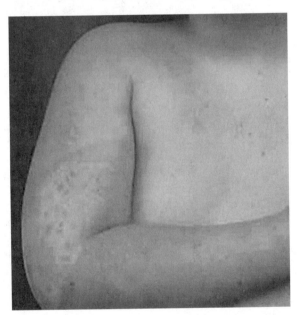

FIG. 12-8. Arm of 7-year-old girl who underwent cadiological ablation procedure with beam positioned laterally, passing through her arm [Vañó E et al.]. Figure also appears in Color Figure section.

Personnel

Cases 1 and 2

Mirhan Krikor Kassabian was one of the first radiologists who intensely investigated the medical utility of fluoroscopy around 1900. He frequently inserted his hands in the direct X-ray beam. Figure 12-9 demonstrates the condition of his hands at the age of 33 years, about 7 years after he started his work with fluoroscopy. He eventually lost fingers on one of his hands and developed

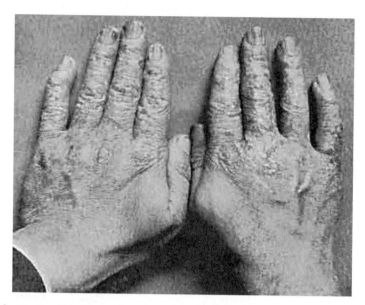

FIG. 12-9. Hands of Mirhan Krikor Kassabian. Age 33 years and about 7 years after starting work with fluoroscopy [Kassabian MK]. Figure also appears in Color Figure section.

radiation-induced cancer, from which he later died at the age of 39. Because of his experiences, Dr. Kassabian was an advocate of learning how to prevent these injuries in beginners.

This historical experience is not just of academic interest. In 1997, the author of this chapter witnessed hands of a pain interventionalist with radiation-induced dermatitis of a striking similarity to that shown in Figure 12-9. These changes developed after several years of constantly inserting his hands into the direct entrance beam of the fluoroscope. Three and a half years after he started his practice, he learned that his condition was radiation dermatitis. His fingernails showed the same brown striations as observed in Dr. Kassabian, and the skin on the backs of his hands was thin and atrophied, with a propensity for slow healing after injury from minor abrasions. The demarcation from healthy to affected skin was pronounced.

The pain interventionalist was taught to use the fluoroscope in a manner inconsistent with good radiation management practice. Proper training in the safe uses of the fluoroscope is essential if physicians are to avoid such injuries.

Case 3

Another physician who performed interventional pain management procedures for several years noticed that the collagen in his hands seemed to be deficient. When held up to a strong light, his hands appeared somewhat translucent. He attributed this to the radiation exposure he experienced over years of work. He then changed his habits and stopped putting his hands in the direct beam. About 10 years later, his hands had recovered mostly from the effects, but atrophy starting in the forearm and extending outward was still apparent along with areas of depigmentation (Fig. 12-10).

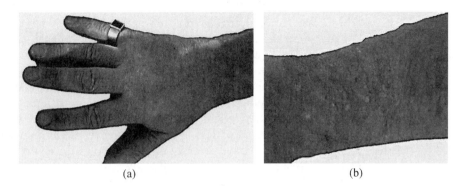

(a)   (b)

FIG. 12-10. **Hand and arm of a pain management interventionalist.** This individual has been in practice for more than 20 years (digitally enhanced to demonstrate radiation induced changes) [Photo supplied by Balter]. Figures also appear in Color Figure section.

Physicians who perform procedures requiring the frequent insertion of hands in or near the direct X-ray beam must learn how to avoid entrance beam irradiation of their hands by working on the exit-beam side of the patient and using mechanical aids and shields. Frequently inserting hands into the direct entrance beam will swiftly lead to doses that are beyond limits recommended by international experts and may place the hands at risk for severe skin damage.

Case 4

Figure 12-11 shows the legs of a 76-year-old interventionalist after 40 years of performing three to six procedures per week. A clear difference in leg-hair growth above and below a line that represents the terminus of the lead apron is evident. The effect was first noticed after 20 years of work. Traumatic contusions in the left leg healed with a pigmented cast.

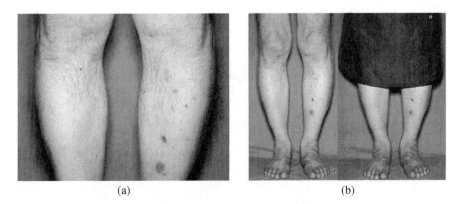

(a)   (b)

FIG. 12-11. **Legs of an interventionalist after 40 years of practice.** Note the distinct line of hair loss below the lead apron [Photo supplied by subject]. Figures also appear in Color Figure section.

With a conventional angiographic unit, wherein the X-ray tube is positioned under the patient with the image intensifier above, backscatter off the underside of the table of the patient is 3–10 times more intense than scatter above the patient. The unprotected portions of the physicians' legs receive a far higher scatter radiation dose than any other portion of the body.

Physicians who perform heavy workloads of interventional fluoroscopy should be aware that there might be long-term effects associated with chronic exposure of their unprotected legs and feet. Many reports of hair loss in the legs of interventionalists have recently surfaced along with reports of changes in skin color. None of these reports identifies any effects of a particularly deleterious nature, but this should serve as a warning bell. With the changes and the increases in interventional work, new generations of physicians will likely be exposing themselves to far greater levels of X rays, with concomitant increases in risk. Designing protection for their legs and feet early in their career is the only sure way to prevent long-term complications in the future.

Cases 5–8

Vañó and co-workers reported on four cases of radiation-induced cataracts in medical personnel involved in interventional procedures that used an overhead X-ray tube. The individuals used no facial shielding and did not wear radiation monitors. After several years of working under these conditions, these four individuals were diagnosed with cataracts that originated in the posterior pole of the lens, consistent with radiation-induced cataract (Fig. 12-12). The chronic exposures to the lens were sufficient to surpass thresholds necessary to cause such an effect. With the beam originating from above the patient, the faces of the medical personnel were subjected to the more intense backscatter radiation from the surface of the patient. A separate case of radiation-induced cataracts in an interventionalist, induced under similar circumstances, is known to these authors.

Training in and execution of the proper use of equipment are essential for good radiation management.

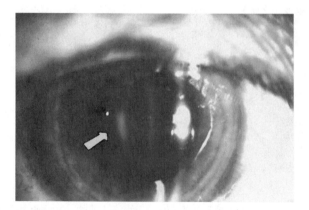

FIG. 12-12. Radiation-induced cataract in an interventional fluoroscopist (arrow) [Vañó E et al.]. Figure also appears in Color Figure section.

MINI COURSE

Long irradiation times place patients at risk for skin injury.

Prolonged irradiation of the same skin area should be avoided when possible.

Irradiation of large patients and through thick body parts markedly increases intensity of exposure at the skin.

The separator cone is essential for radiation safety. If missing, the physician must avoid the hazards that can be encountered by positioning patient skin too close to the port of the X-ray source.

Patients should be screened for previous interventional procedures. If so, it is recommended that the patient be examined for skin changes that would indicate that the skin has less tolerance for further irradiation. Counseling the patient about the situation and avoiding further irradiation of that site are appropriate actions.

Patients should be screened for diseases that might reduce the patient's tolerance to radiation exposure. Such patients should be advised of increased risk in the event that the procedure is prolonged.

Physicians should understand the operation of the specific equipment with which they work so that dose-abating settings can be appropriately employed. This enhances protection for themselves and other personnel and patients.

Direct irradiation of extraneous body parts, such as the arms and female breast, should be avoided by positioning them away from the beam.

Physicians should avoid direct irradiation of their hands.

Physicians who perform large volumes of procedures should be aware of the potential for high exposures to their legs and feet and take appropriate protective measures.

13

Stray Radiation

THE NATURE OF STRAY RADIATION

Stray radiation in the laboratory is undesirable because it contributes to the irradiation of the patient or staff without contributing to the image. Stray radiation is composed of leakage from the X-ray tube and scatter from the patient and from objects in the room. Scatter is the dominant source of stray radiation in fluoroscopy and fluorography. Primary radiation falling outside of the usable X-ray beam is another contributor to unnecessary exposure.

Figure 13-1 illustrates these points in a historical content. The patient's foot is fluoroscoped using an unshielded X-ray tube. The imaging device is a cryptoscope. This device is a simple fluorescent screen enclosed in a dark housing. Perhaps the cryptoscope portrayed in the photograph had a lead-glass primary barrier between the fluoroscopic screen and the operator. In addition, one wonders whether the operator was dark adapted (see Chapter 5).

Radiation leaves the unshielded X-ray tube in virtually all directions. The only photons that might contribute to the image are located in the cone defined by the focal-spot and the fluoroscopic screen. Photons going in other directions may irradiate either the patient or operator.

The operator is exposed to the primary beam emerging from the X-ray tube and to scatter from the interaction of the primary beam with the patient and with objects in the environment. It is not surprising that many early operators suffered from radiation sequela.

All medical X-ray tubes produced in the last half century are "shockproof" and "rayproof." Shockproof means that the high-voltage electrodes are surrounded by electrical grounds. Rayproof means that radiation shielding is built into the tube housing to control the amount of leakage radiation going in directions other than that of the useful beam. Further details of tube construction are found in Chapter 4.

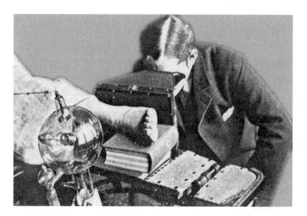

FIG. 13-1. a: Fluoroscopy circa 1910. The operator is using a cryptoscope. Note the lack of radiation shielding and the open high-voltage wire. The figure caption in the original 1915 textbook advised against fluoroscopy.

CONTROL OF THE PRIMARY BEAM

Misaligned collimators are one of the most common findings when testing interventional systems.

In an interventional laboratory, the primary beam should always be confined to the image receptor. In an ideal world, the maximum size and shape of the primary X-ray beam automatically and exactly matches the size and shape of the image receptor (Fig. 13-2). In this ideal world, the operator always manually collimates the beam to the anatomic region of immediate clinical interest.

Real-world conditions, such as the weight of the X-ray tube and image receptor, make this difficult (Fig. 13-3). Regulatory requirements place upper limits on the relative size of the beam. If these tolerances are used, the un-

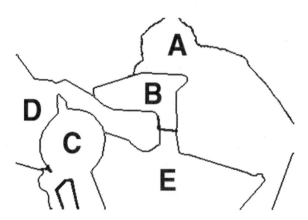

FIG. 13-1. b: Schematic. A: Observer. B: Cryptoscope. C: Unshielded gas X-ray tube. D: Patient. E: Objects contributing to scatter.

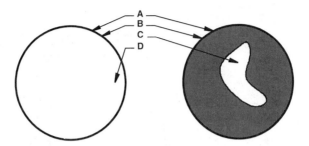

FIG. 13-2. Ideal collimation. A: X-ray beam size does not exceed size of the image receptor. B: Size of the image receptor. C: Collimated to region of interest. D: Collimated to maximum size of the image receptor.

collimated beam is always slightly larger than the active image receptor. This permits full use of the image receptor's field of view. It is also possible to adjust a fluoroscope so that the margins of the primary beam are always fluoroscopically visible. The reduction in the maximum available field of view may or may not be clinically acceptable.

It is both unacceptable and illegal to use a system in which substantial nonvisualized areas are irradiated (Fig. 13-4). This condition can occur if the collimator fails to track changes in source-to-image receptor distance (SID) or the size of the active field of view. Digital magnification of live fluoroscopy is of special importance. Interventional systems should automatically close the X-ray collimator when live digital magnification is used.

The collimator is connected to the SID sensor (Fig. 13-5). This provides full illumination of the image receptor as SID changes. The collimator opens to a wider degree at short SIDs than it does at long SIDs.

PRODUCTION AND DISTRIBUTION OF STRAY RADIATION

The principal sources of stray radiation are leakage from the X-ray tube and scatter from the patient (Fig. 13-6). In most instances, the majority of stray radiation is scatter.

Leakage

A freestanding X-ray tube housing is shielded to limit leakage to a regulatory maximum of 1 mGy/h at 1 meter. This requirement must be met at the maximum operating voltage of the tube (typically 150 kVp). Complete interventional fluoro systems usually have a maximum operating voltage in the range from 100 to 125 kVp. The actual operating voltage is continuously adjusted by the automatic dose-rate control (ADC) circuitry. There will be a workload spectrum of operating voltages dependent on patient size and clinical projection. Tube leakage drops rapidly as the operating kVp decreases. Leakage is negligible, relative to scatter, below 100 kVp. Additional shielding is provided

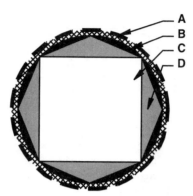

FIG. 13-3. Practical collimation. A: Maximum legal X-ray beam size. B: Active area of the image receptor. C: Largest square field that fits into the image receptor. D: Largest octagonal field. Many collimators use such geometry.

by the heavy metal supports used to attach the X-ray tube to the imaging stand. When these factors are taken into account, it can be seen that tube leakage is likely to be substantially below 1 mGy/h under cardiac fluoroscopic conditions.

Scatter

Reducing scatter increases image quality.

Most of the scatter is produced in the area where the primary X-ray beam enters the patient (Fig. 13-7). Scatter production at fluoroscopic energies is reasonably isotropic and somewhat harder than the primary beam. Thus, the higher primary entrance-beam intensity produces a greater degree of scatter than is produced elsewhere in the patient. Backscatter from the entrance field is minimally attenuated by the patient's tissues.

The spatial distribution of scatter in the laboratory is asymmetric and changes with beam orientation. Most modern interventional systems have two

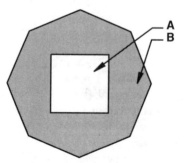

FIG. 13-4. Electronic zoom, without corresponding collimation, is unacceptable. A: Visualized field (defined by image processor). B: Irradiated field (defined by collimator).

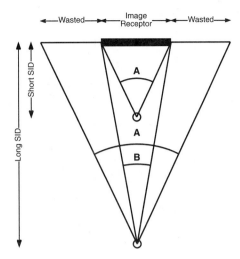

FIG. 13-5. Collimator tracking. The aperture is wider when the SID is short (A) than when it is long. (B).

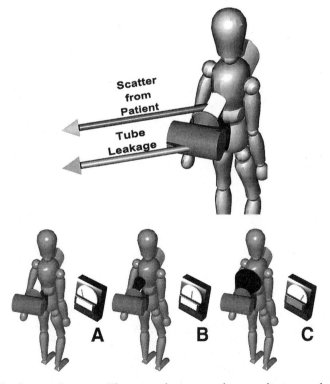

FIG. 13-6. Leakage and scatter. The principle sources of stray radiation are leakage from the X-ray tube and scatter from the patient. In most instances, the majority of stray radiation is composed of scatter. Scatter intensity increases as the X-ray field size increases.

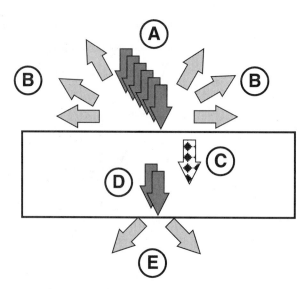

FIG. 13-7. Scatter production vs. depth. A: More intense primary beam on entrance side of phantom. B: More intense scatter on entrance side of phantom. C: Forward scatter attenuated by phantom. D: Attenuated primary beam near exit surface of phantom. E: Less intense scatter on exit side of phantom.

rotational degrees of freedom. (Some systems also have a cradle that permits rotation of the patient around his or her long axis.)

Figures 13-8 to 13-10 illustrate some aspects of the spatial distribution of stray radiation around an interventional system. One can best understand the distribution by remembering that the principal source of stray radiation is scatter from the entrance surface of the patient.

In Figure 13-8, the beam is in a left lateral projection. The entrance field is essentially at the operator's waist level. Figure 13-8a illustrates the isokerma lines describing the intensity of the stray radiation field at 100 cm above the floor (waist level). The X-ray tube is next to the operator. The entrance field is on the patient's side. Backscatter is directed toward the operator's torso and head. This is the worst-case situation in terms of the radiation field at the operator's position. This results in a very high exposure rate at the operator's usual working position (toward the bottom of the drawing). The patient's tissues provide maximum attenuation on the image-intensifier side of the system.

The relative lack of leakage is seen by the shadows in the stray radiation field cast by the X-ray tube in 13-8a. One can also see shadows cast by the image intensifier.

Figure 13-8b illustrates the same projection at 150 cm above the floor (eye level). Exposure rates at this height are reduced by a factor of two on the X-ray tube side. However, less attenuation of scatter by the patient at this height increases the intensity of the stray radiation field on the image-intensifier side.

In the LAO-60 projection (Fig. 13-9), the X-ray tube is still on the operator's side but lower. The beam is angled 60 degrees away from the vertical. The entrance field is under the patient. Backscatter is directed toward the operators lower body and feet.

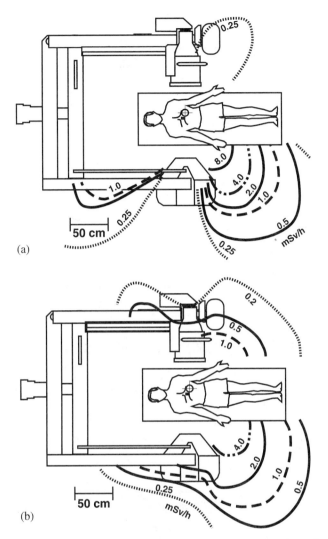

FIG. 13-8. Stray radiation fields for 90° LAO projection. a: 100 cm above the floor. Note the radiation shadow cast by the X-ray tube. b: 150 cm above the floor. The radiation shadow cast by the image intensifier is also evident. Isokerma lines are in units of mSv/h.

In the RAO-30 projection (Fig. 13-10), the X-ray tube is on the opposite side of the patient. The beam is angled 30 degrees away from the vertical. The entrance field is under the patient. Backscatter is directed toward the floor and away from the operator.

These measurements were made with the X-ray beam collimated to the size of the active image intensifier field. The instantaneous scatter rate is proportional to the DAP rate. Many modern cath systems have a built-in dose area product (DAP) meter. It may be useful to note that reducing DAP rate yields a corresponding reduction in the scatter rate everywhere in the lab.

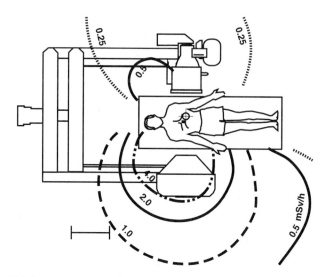

FIG. 13-9. 60° LAO at 100 cm. The maximum scatter intensity at waist level has been reduced by rotating the X-ray tube toward the floor.

Effect of the Asymmetric Field on Personnel Dose Estimates

Fluoroscopists wear protective garments while they move and work in a scatter radiation field that is nonisotropic in both space and time. One needs to interpret the results of film-badge readings with this understanding.

Figure 13-11 illustrates the relative exposures delivered to different parts of the operator's head and body. (The data are normalized to 100 on the

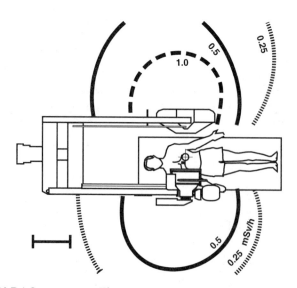

FIG. 13-10. 30° RAO at 100 cm. The maximum scatter intensity is now on the patient's left side. There is a further reduction due to rotating the X-ray tube further toward the floor.

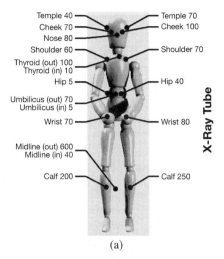

(a)

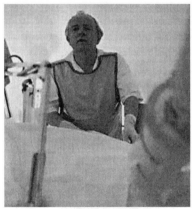

(b)
F. Mason Sones, Jr. M.D.
(Author's Photo c 1976)

FIG. 13-11. Measured relative distribution of exposure. Data have been normalized to 100% for the dosimeter at the thyroid outside the 0.5-mm lead apron (in = inside lead apron, out = outside). The operator is show as seen across the patient table (b). In both cases, the x-ray tube is to the operator's left.

unshielded dosimeter over the thyroid.) These data are the integrated result of 300 complete diagnostic studies performed in 1976 by a pool of 12 experienced operators. The imaging equipment was a U-arm system equipped with fixed collimation confining the beam to a cine frame within the field of view (FOV) of a 6-inch image intensifier. No auxiliary shielding was used during these procedures. The effect of the scatter field gradients is reduced due to operator motion and averaging over all of the projections.

There is a gradient of around 4:1 in the scatter field across the operator. In some cases, the gradient is higher because of shadowing by parts of the imaging equipment or the patient table. Among the lessons that can be learned from these stray radiation measurements is the importance of taking even one step away from the table during fluorography and the variability of film-badge readings solely due to the position where the badge is worn. In addition, shorter operators might be expected to have higher badge readings because they wear their collar badges closer to the patient.

Some clinicians prefer to partially rotate the patient into the beam using a cradle instead of fully rotating the beam around the patient. This tends to direct the backscatter toward the floor. Staff working in "cradle" labs are expected to have lower collar film-badge readings than staff working in the more common "noncradle" labs.

Protective Shielding

Individuals working in an interventional laboratory wear protective garments because they reduce real and perceived radiation risk. In some cases, these garments contain too much lead and are therefore inappropriately heavy. There is a correlation between lead wearing and spinal disk injury. In principle, one could perform an optimization that minimizes both radiation and orthopedic risks.

Movable shielding provides radiation shadows for the staff. These include table-mounted lead flaps, ceiling-mounted face shields, and floor-mounted mobile devices. These shields provide their greatest effect when they are close to the patient and block the line of sight to the beam's entrance point. It is often possible to totally shield the operator from the beam for pure axial beams. This is shown in Figure 13-12. Cranial angulations bring the X-ray tube toward the

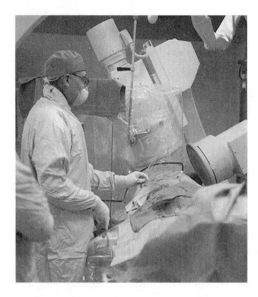

FIG. 13-12. Optimum use of movable radiation protection. The ceiling-mounted shield is perpendicular to and in contact with the patient. A floor shield (seen behind the operator) increases the shadowed zone. Also, note that the patient is in an angulated cradle. [Author's photo]

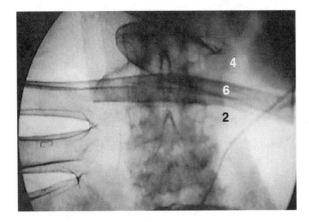

FIG. 13-13. No bony fingers. Fluoroscopic screen shot obtained through a cadaver shows penetration of leaded surgical gloves by radiation. Two layers of glove material are shown on the bottom of the picture, four at the top, and six at the overlap. The system's automatic dose-rate control increased output until the gloves were penetrated.

operator. This motion tends to displace the shielding. Providing an appropriate shield between the patient's entrance surface and the operator without interfering with the examination is an ongoing design challenge.

Commercially available leaded gloves offer limited protection from scatter. Some operators presume that lead gloves allow unlimited hand time in the primary beam. Unfortunately, this is not true. Interventional systems provide automatic dose-rate control. When the glove is in the measuring field, the system simply produces enough output to penetrate it. The sensor sees two layers of lead; the operators' hands are only protected by one. This effect is illustrated in Figure 13-13. The irradiated but unseen field presents a different hazard. Working "just outside" of the field can expose the operator's fingers to primary entrance or exit beams as well as to scatter. Wrist or ring monitors may not "see" this additional exposure.

"No Bony Fingers" is a reminder that it is inappropriate to see a staff member's hands on the monitor.

MINI COURSE

Stray radiation is composed of scatter and leakage. Scatter usually dominates.

The distribution of stray radiation in an interventional lab varies in space and time during a procedure.

Protective shielding significantly attenuates the stray radiation field.

14

Operational Radiation Safety

The goal of any safety program is that of facilitating useful activities while simultaneously reducing the participants' risks to an acceptable level. Achieving this goal requires a balance between the value of the activity and the associated risks. For example, a firefighter will usually enter a burning building to rescue a trapped child. The same firefighter might try to retrieve the child's cat. It is unlikely that an attempt would be made to retrieve the child's lunch.

All activities involve a variety of risks. In many cases, reducing one risk increases another. Achieving a balance between various risks and the benefits of the activity is "relatively" simple when the risks and benefits are all attributable to the same individual. The balance is much more difficult when one person assumes the risks and another person collects the benefits. For example, although the firefighter takes the risk of entering the burning building, the child benefits from being rescued.

Putting a hand into a fire is not risky; this action will certainly produce a burn. Random processes are fundamental to the concept of risk. The magnitudes of some risks (e.g., losing a bet based on a coin toss) are calculated using the laws of probability. Other risks (e.g., being killed by lightning next year) are estimated using statistical tools.

Too high a level of fixed radiation protection is not terribly compatible with the requirement for close access to the patient.

AS LOW AS REASONABLY ACHIEVABLE (ALARA)

What is a "reasonable" level of radiation? Any dose is presumed to carry some risk under the no-threshold assumption. Regulatory authorities set the "maximum permissible doses" (MPD) so that the risk of working with radiation at this level is comparable to the risks of other "safe" occupations. Given what is now known about radiation risks, an individual receiving the MPD every year during an entire working career has no greater risk of dying from a radiation-induced injury than a store clerk has of dying from a store-related injury. (Interventionists seldom accumulate more than a small part of the MPD.)

Eliminating invasive and nuclear procedures reduces occupational exposure of staff members. This is not reasonable from a patient's point of view. Eliminating lead aprons in the interventional lab increases staff dose by a factor of 10 or more. This is not reasonable from the worker's point of view.

BASIC PRINCIPLES

Prudent workers in well-designed interventional labs usually meet the requirements of ALARA. Certain aspects of radiation protection are determined by the design of the room and its equipment. ALARA is largely dependent on staff members habitually doing those things that minimize radiation risk.

The conventional radiation safety triad of principles is "distance," "time," and "shielding." Two additional principles applicable in the interventional lab are "beam management" and "situational awareness."

Beam Management

The primary operator controls the output and direction X-ray beam. Both patient and staff risk are proportional to the total amount of X-ray energy emerging from the tube. The operator can reduce the intensity of the stray radiation field by collimating the beam to less than the full field of view. The stray radiation field changes in shape and intensity as a function of beam direction. This has an important influence on staff risk.

It is worth repeating that there is no risk when the X-ray tube is off. The operator should only produce X-rays when new medically necessary information is needed. Tools such as last-image hold and instant replay have been of considerable help in reducing continuing fluoroscopy while deciding what to do next. A switch to disable X-ray production (while maintaining the remaining functions of the imaging equipment) is prudent. Use of the X-ray disable control eliminates the danger of inadvertent radiation during medical emergencies, room changeover, and so forth.

The traditional cardiac-cath lab provides fluoroscopy (continuous or pulsed) and cinefluorography as the only two modes of operation. There is roughly a 1:10 ratio of output rates between these too modes. This is reasonable for a diagnostic study in which fluoroscopy is used to guide the procedure and cinefluorographic films are later studied to reach a clinical conclusion.

The interventional radiology lab usually offers fluoroscopy, unsubtracted-fluorography, and digital subtracted angiography (DSA). A single DSA frame can require more than 100 times the detector dose of a single fluoroscopic frame. It is important to keep this in mind when using multiple, long, DSA runs.

Interventional procedures require enough image quality for decision making in the lab. Conventional fluoroscopic quality may not be sufficient. Cine quality may be too much. Intermediate dose modes can provide the necessary flexibility. These modes go by any one of a number of occasionally misleading commercial trade names. They provide a substantial decrease in dose rate in comparison to cine. High-dose-rate fluoroscopy without recording the images, *and making use of the data*, is not acceptable. The operator should use these higher dose modes only with instant replay. This provides access to high-quality images while deciding what to do next without continuously irradiating the patient.

Situational Awareness

Supporting staff members need to know when the X-ray beam is active. It is also important to know whether the beam is at fluoroscopic or fluorographic intensity. This is not as easy as it was in former times. At present, images are always visible on the main monitor. It can be difficult to tell at a glance whether these images are live, last-image-hold, or looped playback. Sound may no longer be a clue. Some X-ray tubes rotate continuously and silently. The generator might be installed in a soundproof enclosure. Digital acquisition eliminates mechanical camera sounds. X-ray "active" warning lights need to be visible anywhere in the laboratory. Sound alerts are proposed to indicate fluorographic levels. Perhaps these audio signals could be synthesized rotor or camera sounds.

The region between the X-ray tube and the patient is a danger zone (Fig. 14-1). There is always the chance that the operator might insert a body part into the primary beam. In addition, scattered radiation from the patient is at its most intense in this region. In the region beyond the patient, the patient's tissue attenuates most of the primary and scattered radiation. In this zone, the patient serves as part of the staff's shielding.

Interventional laboratory doors should *not* be equipped with radiation interlocks. These interlocks disable X-ray production when the door is open. This is a dangerous thing to happen in the middle of an intervention. Radi-

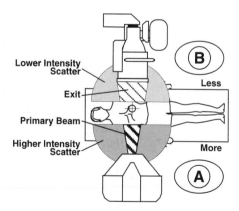

FIG. 14-1. The space between the X-ray tube and the patient is a danger zone. It contains the primary beam and the high-intensity scatter zone. The space between the patient and the image intensifier is less dangerous. It contains the low-intensity exit beam and the lower intensity scatter zone. The individual in position "A" is in a higher radiation field than the individual in position "B." Where possible, work on the image-intensifier side of the patient.

ation warning lights, both inside and outside the room, serve to alert staff to the presence of radiation. Even with lights available, staff members should assume that the beam might be active and take proper precautions whenever they enter the lab.

The operator should refrain from fluoroscopy (and acquisitions) if their hands, or those of their assistants, are in the beam. This happens far too often to be justified as a medical necessity. "No Bony Fingers" is a simple rule to remind staff that their hands should not be seen on the monitor or film.

Distance

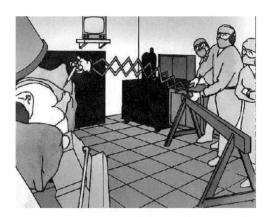

Maintaining an appropriate distance from sources of radiation is an important part of operational radiation protection. The inverse square law states that doubling the distance from a point source of radiation reduces the intensity by a factor of four. Figure 14-2 illustrates this effect. Moving from 1 to 2 m from the point source reduces the intensity from 100 to 25 mGy/h (a reduction by a factor of 4). Moving from 4 to 5 m from the source reduces the intensity from 6.25 to 4 mGy/h. Here, the reduction is a factor of 1.5.

The patient's entrance surface is the source of most of the scattered radiation in the interventional lab. The typical 100-cm² fluoro entrance field is larger than a mathematical point. The exposure reaching any given point on the operator can be calculated using the inverse square law at each point in the field and integrating over the entire field.

Assuming that the entire scatter is emitted from a point in the center of the field is a reasonable approximation at distances greater than four or five times the field diameter.

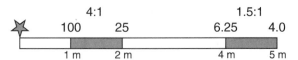

FIG. 14-2. **The reduction factor for dose rate caused by a step back is greater when the starting point is closer to the source.** The star represents a point source. The numbers above the ruler are dose rates. The ratios indicate the reduction in dose rate when moving from 1 to 2 m and from 4 to 5 m, respectively.

Staff members can work in a lower radiation field by maintaining distance from the table. Individuals who do not need to touch the patient while the beam is on should try to stay several steps away from the table. Color coding the floor can be of help (e.g., keep off the gray tiles). The operator can gain a measure of protection by leaning away from the patient.

The author investigated one interventional lab in which the nursing staff had unusually high film-badge readings. This laboratory was just wide enough to swing the gantry. There was no place to retreat. Physically large laboratories provide additional intrinsic radiation protection by simply allowing more distance from the table.

Distance also enters in another manner. Excessive distance between the patient and image intensifier requires increased X-ray output. This unnecessarily increases both patient and staff dose.

In some circumstances, geometric magnification is a clinical necessity. Magnification requires a large spacing between the patient and image receptor. This does increase skin dose relative to the nonmagnification technique. However, it is often possible to remove the grid during a magnification study. Grid removal reduces skin dose. The net increase or decrease in skin dose will depend on individual conditions.

Time

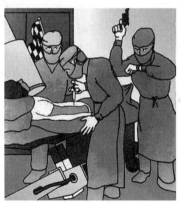

Time as a radioprotective point in the interventional lab has two aspects. These are the operator's control of the beam and the time that staff members occupy high-radiation areas.

X-ray machines produce no radiation when they are off. In general, fluoroscopy is only indicated when the operator needs to observe motion (anatomic, contrast flow, or device placement). Most current systems are equipped with last-image hold and instant-replay features. These images permit clinical decision making without the need for additional radiation and contrast injections.

The operator can often minimize ancillary staff exposure by not fluoroscoping when an assistant needs to be close to the patient. There are occasions when this is not possible. Patient care should be choreographed so that the involved individual moves in, does what has to be done, and moves away as soon as practicable. The choreography should include an approach from the image intensifier side of the system whenever possible.

Remaining in the interventional laboratory without clinical duties is poor practice. Staff members and visitors should refrain from this whenever possible. Appropriate laboratory design facilitates remote observation of the procedure and communication with the clinical team. Architectural details include generously sized control rooms, large viewing windows, supplementary video viewing, and excellent intercom systems.

The five-minute audible timer is more than an annoyance. It is intended to keep the operator aware of the passage of radiation over time.

Shielding

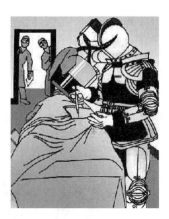

Protective shielding attenuates the radiation field. This reduces the radiation risk of shielded individuals. An appropriate selection and use of shielding balances the radioprotective effects of shielding devices against possible increases in other risks. Shielding may be divided into three classes: structural, movable, and personal. These are ideally mixed and matched to optimize radiation protection.

Structural Shielding

Figure 14-3 illustrates a typical radiation protection plan. The description of the room and its surroundings serves as the basis for calculations.

The radiation protection world is divided into two regions. These are called "controlled" and "noncontrolled" areas. Normally, only radiation workers and patients are permitted in controlled areas. Anyone, including members of the public, is permitted to occupy a noncontrolled area.

Structural shielding barriers are incorporated in the walls, doors, floor, ceiling, and windows. The amount of shielding is designed to reduce the amount of radiation penetrating the barrier to an acceptable level. The calculations, done by the medical physicist or other qualified expert, include considerations of the nature of the proposed equipment and procedures, the anticipated workload of the laboratory, the occupancy of adjacent areas, and other factors.

To repeat, a well-shielded and amply sized control room encourages observers to stay outside of the lab. The provision of a large window and a good intercom is in keeping with the ALARA philosophy.

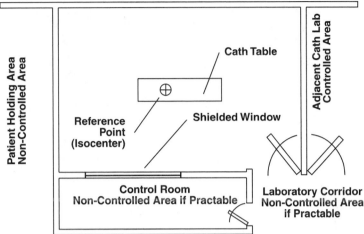

FIG. 14-3. Example of information needed for a radiation protection plan. The required structural shielding is a function of both the volume and nature of procedures in the room and on the individuals expected to be found in the surroundings. Where practicable, the control room and corridor should be designed as noncontrolled areas.

In most cases, protective barriers allow nonradiation workers into the control room and other adjacent spaces. However, the original design of a laboratory may have been based on special assumptions. It is prudent to check with the qualified expert before allowing substantial changes of activities in the immediate vicinity of a lab.

Mobile fluoroscopic imaging systems may be capable of supporting many invasive procedures. However, wheels do not provide a radioprotective effect. The neighbors of any room in which such equipment is routinely used are entitled to appropriate structural shielding.

Movable Shielding

A great variety of ceiling-, table-, and floor-mounted shields can be found in and around an interventional lab. All too often, these "gadgets" are stored in a corner so that they "do not get in the way of the procedure." Perhaps their usage will increase when laboratory staff members realize that mobile shielding can reduce the required weight of lead aprons.

Shielding casts a protective shadow. As shown in Figure 14-4, the size of the protected zone increases when the shielding is moved closer to the source of radiation. In the interventional lab, small movable shields are most effective when they are placed close to the patient.

Large shields also have a place because they cast a larger shadow. The additional bulk of such shields is warranted when small shields unduly restrict access to the patient.

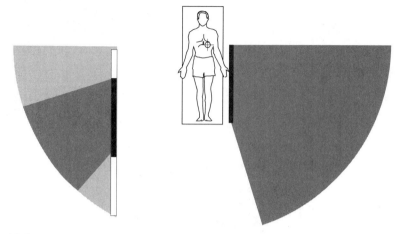

FIG. 14-4. Shadow shield. A radiation shield casts a protective shadow. The size of the shielded zone is increased when the shield is close to the patient. Large remote shields may be needed for patient access.

All shielding devices should be placed so that they block the line of sight from the entrance port of the X-ray beam (on the patient) to the shielded staff member.

Personal Shielding

Lead Apron

The lead apron is the interventionalist's badge of office. Proper use of this and other types of protective clothing can reduce effective dose, and hence radiation risk, to an acceptably low level. Overshielding may increase the risk of musculoskeletal injury or may impede patient access. In some cases, massive personal shielding impedes access to and communication with the patient.

It is not a surprise that the shielding element in most "lead aprons" is lead itself. The typical lead thickness is 0.5 mm. In some locations, local regulations require this thickness as a minimum.

The K absorption edge of lead, at 69 keV, is higher than the energy of much of the scatter present in the cath lab. Lower atomic number elements, such as tin (K edge = 29 keV), have higher mass attenuation coefficients than lead for scatter over much of the scatter spectrum. Where appropriate, shielding made of tin or similar materials provide equivalent attenuation with less weight. Tin is less efficient than elemental lead for softer and harder spectra. The choice of shielding material should be made after considering typical X-ray factors in your laboratory.

Well-fitted aprons provide a barrier between the radiation source and the wearer's tissue. (The main source of scattered radiation in the interventional lab is the beam entry port into the patient.) Frontal aprons are useful when the wearer faces the source. Wrap-around clothing provides protection in any orientation. Shielding is compromised if the armholes are too wide.

The choice of one-piece or two-piece construction is a matter of individual anatomy and preference. The two-piece style takes much of the weight off the operator's shoulders. It does require a body shape that would keep the kilt portion in place with minimum discomfort.

Thyroid Collar

The thyroid collar is a logical extension of the lead apron. Shielding the thyroid yields a significant reduction in Effective Dose with little inconvenience to the wearer. An appropriate thickness is 0.5 mm lead (equivalent).

Lead aprons and thyroid collars are subject to wear. Outer layers of fabric usually cover the lead-bearing layer. Damaged lead may not be visually identifiable. Lead garments need to be fluoroscoped annually to verify their integrity. The institution's radiation safety officer normally does this. The apron can be fluoroscoped at any time if there is any doubt about its integrity. Small holes, such as from stitching, can be ignored. Larger holes, tears, or missing panels are causes for rejecting the apron.

Leaded Surgical Gloves?

Leaded surgical gloves are available on the market. Depending on the model, these provide an attenuation factor ranging from 5 to 20%. This may or may not be of some benefit when the operator's hands are out of the direct beam. In some instances, the lessened tactile sensitivity when wearing these gloves actually prolongs procedures and hence total hand dose.

Leaded surgical gloves are contraindicated when the operator's hand is in the X-ray beam. When a hand encased in a leaded glove is in the beam, the X-ray system's automatic dose rate control will increase the output until the gloved hand is penetrated. Radiation output is increased enough to penetrate two layers of glove material; the hand is protected by only one layer of the same material. Seeing one's hand on the monitor or on a fluorographic recording is usually evidence of poor procedure.

NO BONY FINGERS: It is poor practice to see staff hands in the image.

Leaded Eye Glasses?

The lens of the eye is relatively insensitive to radiation. Radiogenic cataracts are deterministic injuries with a single fraction threshold of 2 Gy. Fractionating radiation over a month increases the threshold to around 5 Gy. The maximum permissible dose (MPD) for X-ray exposures of the eye is 0.15 Gy per year. An individual would need to accumulate the eye MPD over more than 30 years to reach the cataract threshold. This is virtually impossible for operators of systems with undertable X-ray tubes. However, cataracts have been reported in interventional laboratories with overtable X-ray tubes.

Shielded lenses are not especially helpful in the cath lab. Nevertheless, eye protection against liquid splatter is recommended as a part of universal precautions. Adding radiation shielding may increase the operator's comfort level. Two factors need to be considered if an individual chooses to wear "lead glasses." Side shields are needed because the direct line from the patient's entrance port to the operator's eye seldom passes through the normal eyeglass lens. The glasses need to be certified as shatter resistant to minimize the probability of eye damage due to a mechanical accident.

Don't Panic

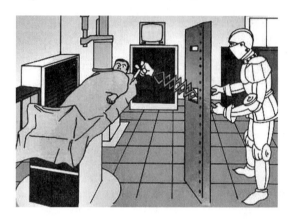

Radiation is only one of the risks to which cath lab staff is exposed. Good radiation-safety habits do not impose a huge intellectual or physical workload on the staff. Prudent staff members can reduce their effective dose well below the 10 mSv/year MPD. Indeed, the effective dose of everyone except the primary operator is usually less than 1 mSv/year. This latter value is the difference in the effective dose attributable to natural background radiation when living in New York or living in Denver. With prudent care, the primary operator's effective dose seldom exceeds a few mSv/y. These values comply with the ALARA concept. Beyond this point, available resources might better be expended to minimize nonradiation risks. The balanced approach maximizes total safety.

MINI COURSE

Distance
Time
Shielding
Beam Management
Situational Awareness

15

Radiation Safety Regulations and Requirements

INTRODUCTION

Radiation is a highly feared environmental pollutant. Public apprehension about the dangers of radiation and other pollutants is real. The word "radiation" evokes images of atomic bombs, nuclear power plant accidents, and other disasters. Opinions are often formed on the basis of dramatic incidents that have been portrayed by the media. Fear often leads to political demands that the risk be totally eliminated. The legislative and regulatory processes need to be responsive to both political demands for absolute safety and the social need for the beneficial uses of radiation. The administration of these programs is based on a legislatively approved health code. Public apprehension about radiation tends to mold conservative regulations.

There was zero risk from the deliberate medical use of X-rays in 1894 (the year before Roentgen's discovery). One way to eliminate the largest single cause of human made exposure is to outlaw the medical use of radiation. From a patient perspective, this is not a good idea. Few will argue that the availability of X-rays has been remarkably beneficial. The challenge is to use radiation in a way that maximizes benefits to the patient without exposing either patients or staff to unnecessary risk. There have been excesses. For example, many shoe stores offered fluoroscopy in the 1940s and 1950s. Shoe-fitting fluoroscopes irradiated many people without any real benefit. These devices have since been banned.

Given that some uses of radiation are beneficial, the essential element of a radiation safety program is that the benefits outweigh the risks. Three distinct risk groups need to be considered. The first are patients who are exposed to radiation for diagnosis or treatment. The radiation risks in this group are directly born by the radiation beneficiaries. The second group is comprised of radiation workers (such as X-ray technologists). These individuals are presumed to accept the risks of working with radiation in exchange for the benefits of their employment. In some cases, radiation workers will accept greater personal risk from the radiation in exchange for delivering better care to their patients. The third group is the public. These people might be exposed when they are near an active radiation source. There is no individual benefit associated with such exposure. Strategies for radiation protection differ for each of these groups.

Given public opinions about radiation and the limitations of the regulatory process, governmental and institutional radiation protection programs are generally reasonable. Fear of radiation has funneled generous research resources into this area. The effects of radiation are, arguably, the best known of any pollutant. This knowledge, coupled with a deliberately conservative dose-effect model contributes to a safe working environment. The medical radiation risk to workers and the public is stochastic and usually a small fraction of the risk from natural background radiation. Judgment is needed to achieve a consensus on just what is an acceptable risk.

Radiation protection recommendations in the 1930s were given in terms of a tolerance dose. In 1934, the recommended tolerance dose in the United States (approximately 300 mSv/year in today's units) was half the international level. This was considered a safe level of exposure even when sustained over a working lifetime. It is also interesting to note that the values were based on 300 working days per year! Although these levels are very high by today's recommendations (lifetime average below 10 mSv/year in the United States), they were low enough to eliminate most occupational radiation injuries.

Current radiation protection regulations are designed to limit the stochastic risk of radiation-induced cancer or genetic disease. It is not surprising to find that different groups of experts draw somewhat different conclusions from the same data. Implementation differences are more reflective of intellectual diversity than of fundamental disagreement. There are sufficient common data to conclude that the scientific and operational basis of radiation protection is on reasonably solid ground.

Most radiation workers receive zero occupational dose. Interventionalists receive a few mSv or less per year.

COMMITTEES AND COMMISSIONS

The scientific basis of radiation protection has been collected into two series of reports. One of these is published by the United Nations Scientific Commission on the Effects of Atomic Radiation (UNSCEAR). The second such series comes from the United States National Academy of Science. Its title is *Biological Effects of Ionizing Radiation* (BEIR). A report in each series is expected in the next few years.

Both sets of reports include and evaluate evidence of radiation effects attributable to natural background, nuclear weapons, medical exposures, and other radiation sources. Virtually all of the evidence regarding low-level exposures are statistical in nature. The error bars are large. As might be expected, UNSCEAR and BEIR do not use exactly the same data or reach exactly the same conclusions. Nevertheless, the maximum credible risk attributable to occupational-level radiation exposure is low.

Operational aspects of radiation protection also appear in two distinct flavors. These are published by the International Commission on Radiation Protection (ICRP) and by the United States National Commission on Radiation Protection and Measurements (NCRP). These series also contain a great deal of background (forgive the pun) and reference information.

The International Commission on Radiological Units (ICRU) was established in 1925 at the first meeting International Congress of Radiology in London. The objective of the ICRU was to define a standard method for measuring the "amount" of radiation.

The ICRP had its first meeting in 1928. It was able to use the ICRU's definition of the Roentgen as a means of describing radiation fields. The ICRP's initial recommendations on radiation safety (for X rays and radium) predate the nuclear era by almost 30 years.

Several United States professional societies organized an "Advisory Committee on X-ray and Radium Protection" in 1929. Its initial mission was to develop medical radiation protection safety standards for the US. Over time, the organization's mission has been broadened and its name changed to the United States National Council on Radiation Protection and Measurements. The early NCRP abbreviation established in the 1950s has survived the expansion of the organization's formal name.

Both the ICRP and NCRP review and use UNSCEAR and BEIR data as part of the scientific basis of their reports. The NCRP series serve as the basis for many United States regulations. ICRP reports have their greatest influence elsewhere in the world. The general flow of recommendations is similar in both sets of reports. As might be expected, there are differences in detail, emphasis, and numerical values. Interventional equipment is usually built for a world market. These systems usually conform to both NCRP and ICRP requirements.

The International Electrotechnical Commission (IEC) is a voluntary international standards organization. Its emphasis is on the construction and functional aspects of electrical equipment such as X-ray systems. There is an increasing focus on equipment aspects of radiation safety. IEC standards are increasingly adopted as regulatory requirements by both the European Union (EU) and the United States Food and Drug Administration (FDA).

REGULATORY FRAMEWORK

Maximum Permissible Dose, ALARA—NCRP

Radiation management programs were originally based on the concept of tolerance. Dose limits were originally expressed in terms of "tolerance dose" because it was believed that a worker could tolerate such a dose without injury. This was appropriate in a time when all radiation injuries were assumed to have a threshold (deterministic injury). Some early radiation protection regulations specified double vacations for radiation workers. It is not certain whether this was done as a protection against radiation, ozone from the open electrical systems of the time, or exposure to photographic chemicals. It is sad to report that last of these regulations disappeared in the 1980s.

By the early 1950s, it was recognized that there were two broad classifications of radiation effects. These are deterministic injury and stochastic risk. Deterministic injury occurs when the dose is high enough to cause massive cell killing. Radiation protection limits against deterministic effects are set well below the known thresholds. Stochastic risk relates to the chance that a dose of radiation will cause inheritable genetic damage or the production of a malignant change in a cell.

Radiobiology teaches that there is a latent period of years to decades between the induction of a malignancy in a single cell and its expression as a clinical cancer. Epidemiological research reveals many environmental carcinogenic factors. It is impossible to directly correlate cause and effect at dose levels comparable with or below those experienced by interventional fluoroscopists.

The current NCRP radiation risk model assumes that stochastic risk is proportional to a lifetime accumulation of dose. Repair of radiation effects is presumed to be nonexistent. The model assumes that there is some small probability that a single X-ray photon could induce a malignant change. This conservative model is called the linear no-threshold model (LNT).

Absolute dose limits cannot logically exist in the LNT model. The establishment of regulatory dose limits for stochastic events is arbitrary. Levels are based on judgments of relative risk and the availability of economic resources. Levels for the public are set at a fraction of occupational levels.

Current NCRP recommendations are shown in Table 15-1. This table tabulates the maximum permissible dose (MPD) for various circumstances. The MPD for deterministic effects are set below known biological thresholds. For example, the MPD for the lens of the eye is 150 mSv/y. This leads to a maximum eye dose of 6,000 mSv for a 40-year career. The known threshold for radiation-induced lens opacities is 2,000 mSv in a single exposure and 4,000

TABLE 15-1. Maximum permissible doses[1] [from NCRP 116]

	Occupational exposures
Whole-body exposures: effective dose limits	
Annual	50 mSv/yr
Cumulative	10 mSv × age (yr)
Partial body: equivalent dose annual limits for tissues and organs	
Lens of Eye	150 mSv/yr
Skin, hands, feet	500 mSv/yr
Public exposures: effective dose limit	
Frequent exposures	1 mSv/yr
Infrequent exposures	5 mSv/yr
Fetal dose limit	0.5 mSv/mo

[1]Excluding medical exposures and doses from natural sources.

mSv protracted over 1 month. It is reasonable to assume that there is an additional safety factor with decades of protraction.

The occupational MPDs for stochastic effects are judgment calls designed to provide a safe working environment. Given the LNT model, a dose just above the MPD is only slightly less safe than a dose just below the MPD. Lower is better. The entire radiation protection program is structured to minimize dose. If there really is a linear increase in stochastic risk with dose, it is inappropriate to operate just below the MPD. A major concept is to keep the dose "as low as reasonably achievable" (ALARA). The goal is to minimize dose unless there is a reasonable justification to do otherwise.

There are two stated values for the occupational whole-body dose. The first is a limit of 50 mSv in any one year. The second value is a lifetime accumulation of 10 mSv × age. One should not tap into the unused reserve. Thus, the actual occupational MPD should not exceed 10 mSv per year. This needs to be rephrased using ALARA: The actual occupational MPD should not exceed a fraction of 10 mSv per year.

The "public" whole-body MPD for continuous irradiation is 1 mSv per year. This design principle presumes that there is someone (e.g., a receptionist) always present in a noncontrolled space. Natural background radiation levels increase by more than 1 mSv/year when living in Denver rather than in New York (see Figs. 15-1 and 15-2). Given such background variations, the public MPD is about as low as it can reasonably go.

The public MPD is 5 mSv per year for occasional irradiation. Circumstances in which this applies include family members of a nuclear medicine or radionuclide radiotherapy patient. The fetal exposure limit is based on this concept. The fetus is considered a member of the public who is inadvertently irradiated during the course of the mother's occupation.

In keeping with the spirit of ALARA, many radiation safety officers begin to investigate circumstances when dose exceeds 25% of the MPD. A more rigorous investigation is required at the 50% level. The net effect of the pro-

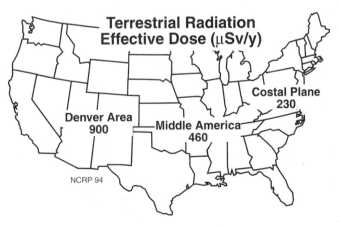

FIG. 15-1. Terrestrial radiation. Levels vary with geological variation in concentration of natural radioactive materials in rock and soil. [Based on NCRP 94]

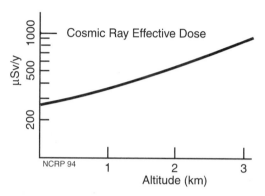

FIG. 15-2. Cosmic radiation. Levels increase with altitude due to less atmospheric shielding. [Based on NCRP 94]

gram is that very few radiation workers receive any significant fraction of the MPD.

Epidemiological studies of large groups of radiation workers have failed to demonstrate increases in disease. Indeed, some of the studies have demonstrated a "healthy worker syndrome." Members of these cohorts are statistically healthier than their counterparts in other occupations. Reasons include a statistical fluctuation, the possible beneficial effect of exposures to low levels of radiation (called hormesis), and job selection bias.

Dose Limits, Justification, and Optimization—ICRP

The ICRP's approach is to set dose limits, justify any level of radiation dose, and a continue optimization of the process to minimize dose. This management process is to use radiation only when appropriate. Dose limits are not permitted levels. Justification includes explaining the reason for any irradiation. Optimization includes a balance between the risks of a particular radiation level and the social and economic costs that need to be expended to reduce the level of radiation. The ICRP's rules are often the basis of governing legislation in much of the world. The requirements are similar for the United States and the European Union. In less developed areas, local justification might allow the use of less expensive technologies rather than pricing radiation imaging beyond the local pocketbook.

Different Aspects of the Same Basic Advice

The bottom line is that radiation is not to be applied to a human being (patient, worker, or member of the public) unless there is a useful purpose. In the simplest terms, radiation is only justified if the person authorizing the use can verbally explain its necessity. (Referring to a routine checklist does not count.) In medical terms, the ordering physician must have an expectation that the information to be gained from the procedure is needed for patient management.

ALARA and optimization both imply that the quantity of radiation be limited. Neither requires that the technologically possible lowest amount of radiation be all that is allowed. It is usually prudent to use somewhat more than the minimum to avoid procedural failure due to insufficient image quality. A usual caveat is that dose should be minimized, "social and economic factors being taken into consideration." A simplified rule is to "waste" as little radiation as is prudent.

Dose limits and MPDs provide administrative levels for managing a radiation protection program. Under both systems, the intent is to lower the risk by lowering the dose. It is not socially acceptable to allow many instances of doses near the limit. As previously noted, an intensive investigation and vigorous dose reduction process is usually triggered at the 50% level.

Patient dose management in diagnostic imaging is beginning to undergo similar scrutiny. The methodology for doing this is discussed in the quality assurance chapter of this book (Chapter 17).

REGULATORY BODIES

In the United States, regulatory authority for X rays is the responsibility of the state health department. Regulatory authority for certain aspects of X-ray equipment performance is assigned to the FDA. Regulatory authority for radionuclides may be either the responsibility of the state (in agreement states) or the United States Nuclear Regulatory Commission (NRC). Because of the differences in the sources of radiation exposure, there are some inconsistencies between X-ray and radionuclide monitoring rules. This chapter mainly discusses X-ray rules and regulations.

The Council of Radiation Control Program Directors (CRCPD) is a voluntary organization composed of senior federal and state radiation officials. It publishes a uniform set of suggested state regulations (SSRs) to help minimize state-to-state inconsistencies. It takes some time for a version of the SSRs to become state policy. This inevitable result is that regulations run behind the best available science.

Federal regulations are part of the United States Code. State regulations are part of individual state health codes. Given regulatory time scales, the desire to have conservative regulations, and the complexity of the underlying science, it is not surprising to find inconsistencies from state to state. Federal rules and regulations, where they exist, take precedence over state regulations.

Codes of regulations are complex documents. They try to anticipate every situation and provide an unambiguous method of compliance. Necessary simplifications often bias the results in a conservative direction. One example of this is the assignment of a transport index (TI) to a package of radioactive material before it is shipped. A fragment from the International Atomic Energy Agency's regulations is shown in the insert. The net result of the process is very useful. The transport index is written on a required radiation label on the package. By adding the TIs of all the packages, a truck driver can easily determine whether or not there is too much radioactive material in the load.

Extract from IAEA Regulations: "The value determined in steps (a) and (b) shall be rounded up to the first decimal place (e.g., 1.13 becomes 1.2, except that a value of 0.05 or less may be considered zero."

PERSONAL DOSIMETRY

Most people are concerned about their personal radiation risk. Appropriate personal radiation monitoring is the only reasonable way to assess the amount of received radiation and hence to assess the risk. There are two major aspects: wearing of the monitors and interpretation of the results.

In the interventional environment, it is recommended that "scrubbed staff" use radiation monitors as shown in Table 15-2. Remaining employees are adequately monitored with a single above-lead monitor. Readings on this latter group are expected to be low.

It is difficult to convince all of the diverse personalities in a laboratory to consistently use their dosimeters. The list of reasons is often longer than the staff roster. One legitimate complaint can be overly conservative regulatory interpretation of the results. For most of the rest, it suffices to say that personal radiation safety is as much a part of good radiation habits as anything else. Without adequate monitoring, it is virtually impossible to identify failing infrastructure or inappropriate habits.

Some jurisdictions still base regulatory decisions on the formal presumption that the whole-body dose is equal to the highest single monitor reading. This can be a problem because cath lab workers wear lead aprons to reduce the risk of working in a radiation field. Monitor interpretations must consider this. The current SSRs provide a procedure for calculating an effective dose equivalent from single- and dual-monitor readings. This reasonable procedure is outlined in Table 15-3.

What does all this mean? Both the single- and double-badge scenarios prescribe locations for wearing the monitors. The single-badge procedure accepts an overestimate at values so far below the whole-body MPD that they are not of regulatory concern. The reading is partially adjusted to account for shielding when it becomes high enough to attract attention. The use of the 0.3 factor in the one-badge method balances the MPDs of the whole-body, eye, and thyroid. The two-badge reading was developed by Webster. This reading accounts for the shielding provided by the lead apron and the thyroid collar. The waist badge reading is increased to account for unshielded body parts. The collar reading is decreased to reflect that there is little tissue at risk

TABLE 15-2. Radiation monitor locations

Body	Midline, waist—under the lead apron
Head	Midline, thyroid—above the lead thyroid collar
Hands	Ring dosimeters, if there is a possibility that the operator's hands might be in the beam

TABLE 15-3. Dose assignment for fluoroscopists[1] [from Suggested State Regulations for the Control of Radiation]

When only one individual monitoring device is used and it is located at the neck outside the protective apron, the reported deep dose equivalent shall be the (H_E) for external radiation; or

When only one individual monitoring device is used and it is located at the neck outside the protective apron, and the reported dose exceeds 25% of the limit specified, the reported deep dose equivalent value, multiplied by 0.3, shall be the (H_E) for external radiation; or

When individual monitoring devices are worn, both under the protective apron at the waist and outside the protective apron at the neck, the (H_E) for external radiation shall be assigned: (H_E) = 1.5 × (waist reading) + 0.04 × (collar reading)[2]

[1]These rules use effective dose equivalent, the NCRP recommendations use effective dose.
[2]The collar reading indicates eye dose.

in the head and neck area. The collar reading is also used to assess the dose received by an unshielded thyroid and by the lens of the eyes.

The latest monitoring recommendations are found in NCRP Report 122. This document contains an extensive analysis of techniques used to evaluate fluoroscopists' radiation monitor readings. The Webster model is accepted for estimating effective dose equivalent (H_E).[1] A separate method is used to estimate effective dose (E). *Note: the NCRP recommendations for whole-body MPD is expressed in terms of effective dose.* The NCRP formula for calculating E is

$$E(1 \text{ badge}) = \text{reading}/21$$
$$E(2 \text{ badge}) = 0.5 \times \text{shielded} + 0.025 \times \text{unshielded}$$

The NCRP report states that for a fluoroscopist wearing a 0.5-mm lead apron, the estimates of E obtained using the two-badge formula ranges from 1.06 to 1.96 times the actual value. The variation is due to differences in X-ray beam quality, patient, and field size.

The two-monitor formula is shown graphically in Figure 15-3. The annual readings of the shielded (waist—under lead) and unshielded (thyroid—over lead) badges are shown on the ordinate and abscissa, respectively. The over-lead reading is cut off at 150 mSv per year. This value corresponds to the MPD for the eye. The under-lead reading should never exceed the over-lead value. When this happens, it is evidence that the badges were switched.

The MPD shown in this chart is an effective dose of 10 mSv per year. It is simply good practice to limit dose accumulation to this rate and not to dip into reserves. The diagonal lines correspond to 10%, 25%, 50%, and 100% of the MPD calculated using the two-badge formula.

The region below the 10% line (lower line) represents an occupational effective dose of less than 1 mSv per year. This corresponds to the difference in natural background radiation between New York and Denver. Occupational

[1]As presently specified in the SSRs.

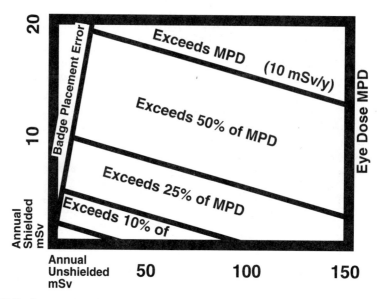

FIG. 15-3. Conversion of annual dose monitor readings to effective dose. See text for explanation. The same chart can be used to interpret monthly or quarterly readings with the use of appropriate scale factors.

dose values in this region should not be of any concern. Most laboratory staff, including a significant fraction of operators, receive doses in this region.

The >10% region represents occupational doses higher than an individual might usually encounter by changing living locations. The radiation risks at this level are generally deemed acceptable. Virtually all high-volume operators are found in this region.

The >25% region begins to attract attention of the radiation safety office. Very few medical radiation workers should routinely occupy this region. In many facilities, such readings usually trigger an investigation. The purpose of the investigation is to devise means for reducing the risk of the affected person.

The >50% region represents a zone that is simply too high for routine medical work. Radiation safety offices aggressively investigate the cause of the dose and then escalate a search for dose reduction.

A medical worker achieving readings exceeding the MPD is in a most unusual situation. Such an individual has now exceeded the formal level of acceptable risk. In many states, the health code requires stopping radiation work when the MPD is exceeded.

Caution: A facility, such as a hospital, and its workers have legal requirements to comply with local regulations. Individual state health codes have different rules for wearing badges and interpreting badge readings, for investigation levels, and for limiting radiation work. This may or may not be a problem for busy operators. However, not wearing badges to avoid administrative hassles removes one of the few available dose reduction feedback mechanisms.

STAFF PREGNANCY

Discussions about radiation management with a pregnant or potentially pregnant worker require more than a marshalling of scientific facts. The maternal protective instinct is strong and, appropriately, difficult to influence. In some instances, facilities are too protective. In such cases, one must take care to comply with pregnancy-related antidiscrimination regulations. In all cases, the need to provide continuity of patient care is also a social necessity. Many factors have to be balanced without placing an unacceptable burden on either the pregnant worker or other staff members.

Most radiation protection regulations are not permitted to consider a woman pregnant until she chooses to make a formal declaration of pregnancy. The usual policy is to issue an abdominal radiation monitor to woman when they declare themselves pregnant. This policy, when coupled with opportunities to discuss concerns with knowledgeable individuals, can be very helpful.

The maximum permissible fetal dose is 5 mSv for the entire pregnancy. To reach this level, a woman would have to receive 1 mSv each month to her abdominal skin (under the lead apron). An additional factor of two is considered to allow for the attenuation of the radiation by the mother's tissues. Very few interventional lab workers, of either gender, have any measurable reading under the apron. In such cases, occupational exposure of a pregnant worker makes a minimal contribution to fetal dose. It is important to investigate the causes of any under-lead reading on a pregnant worker.

Radiation-induced congenital abnormalities are often of concern. In the absence of radiation exposure or other known risk factors, the natural incidence of recognizable abnormalities is around 5% of births. These facts need to be included in radiation safety lectures and reviewed once a worker declares that she is pregnant.

On the basis of studies of the atomic bomb populations, the major deterministic effect of fetal exposure in humans is a reduction in intelligence. This effect is seen for fetal irradiation between *weeks* 8 and *15*. This may be a linear no-threshold effect with an IQ loss of approximately 20 points at 1,000 mSv. This practical threshold is well above the 5-mSv fetal dose limit for the entire pregnancy.

The risk of stochastic injury resulting from exposure of the young requires special attention. In simple terms, a child has a full lifetime to express the results of an injury. Other considerations include differences between adult and fetal or juvenile physiology. Radiation protection regulations reflect these concerns.

PATIENT EXPOSURE

There are no legal limitations on the amount of radiation that may be delivered to patients as part of their medical diagnosis or treatment. The presumption is that the responsible physician concludes that the medical benefits of the procedure will exceed the radiation (and other) risks.

Aspects of this process are the dose needed to form each particular image and the number and type of acquired images. Technological and regulatory constraints can limit the per-image dose. The other two conditions are related to clinical decisions.

There are regulatory limits on fluoroscopic exposure rates. The FDA limit for interventional fluoroscopy is 10 R/min when measured 30 cm in front of the image intensifier. The actual maximum patient skin exposure rate can exceed the regulatory limit if the entrance skin surface is more than 30 cm away from the image intensifier.

There are no present regulatory limits on video, digital, or cine-film acquisitions. Regulatory initiatives might intervene in this situation in the next few years. Less is not always better. Too low an exposure rate might produce unusable images and "waste" all of the radiation.

The total dose received by the patient is determined by the choice of equipment and the operator's choice of imaging modes and operating times. Several interventional procedures (coronary angioplasty, neuroembolization, and radio-frequency catheter ablation) were listed by the FDA in 1994 to be high risks for radiation-induced skin injury. There is no regulatory imperative to always avoid skin injury. In rare cases, it may be impossible to complete a life-saving procedure without inflicting an injury. Such an event should only occur after careful clinical consideration of the situation. Accurate dosimetry is a prerequisite.

Technology exists to estimate the patient's skin dose while the case is in progress. Keeping track of radiation should be as much of the clinical process as keeping track of iodine use. Skin dose meters (not dose-area product meters) are available either built in or added on to the angiographic system. The IEC will soon require built-in dose monitoring on new equipment. Dose monitoring of all intensive interventional procedures is likely to be a regulatory requirement in the next few years.

Pregnant Patients

The pregnant interventional patient is a special concern. The usual cautions against performing elective procedures are especially valid in an interventional fluoro setting. Considerations include the potential effects of pharmaceutical agents as well as ionizing radiation.

Procedures needed to deal with urgent and emergent conditions present a different risk-benefit balance. Under some circumstances, interventional fluoro procedures are better for the mother and fetus than available alternatives. The goal in these cases is to perform the appropriate procedure while minimizing fetal dose.

Direct pelvic irradiation should be avoided whenever possible. Consideration should be given to fluoroscopically blind insertion of devices via a femoral puncture site. Another option is to use a different route of arterial access.

Minimizing dose area product minimizes the production of scatter. This minimizes fetal dose. Pelvic shielding is of value when placed between the X-ray tube and the patient. A shield on the patient's abdomen does not help much if the X-ray tube is under the patient.

It is helpful to discuss the risks and benefits of the procedure as well as dose limiting measures with the patient before beginning the procedure.

TRAINING

Patient and staff exposures are for the most part determined by the way the operator elects to operate the equipment. It is therefore important that operators understand how the equipment operates and the trade-off between radiation and image quality. Acquiring the necessary knowledge requires an appropriate investment in a formal training setting. A radiation license, as evidence of training, is required in a few states and institutions. Appropriate training for all other laboratory staff is also required. This is essential because personal behavior is a major risk-management factor. Training resources are usually available from the radiation safety officer or medical physicist.

It is also important for an operator to understand the operation of each individual angiographic system. This facilitates the use of dose-management elements of the equipment. A 10-minute check ride with an experienced technologist or service engineer is often all that is required.

MINI COURSE

Any use of radiation needs to be justified and optimized.

Radiation safety regulations use conservative scientific models to establish staff and public dose levels.

Staff awareness and training are critical parts of the radiation management program.

16

Endovascular Brachytherapy

INTRODUCTION

Radiation has been used in the treatment of disease for more than a century. It remains one of the procedures of choice for malignancy. Because of the risk of cancer induction, the treatment of benign disease by radiation has been deliberately limited in the past half-century.

Brachytherapy is the placement of sources of radiation in or near the target tissue. The resulting dose distribution is therapeutically high near the sources and rapidly drops elsewhere in the patient. Brachytherapy is usually performed using radioactive materials.

Most of the techniques under investigation involve the endovascular placement of beta- or gamma-emitting radionuclides. Endovascular and external beam X-ray therapies are also to be considered. The eventual optimization includes a delivery system that can deliver appropriate radiation doses to the target tissues while simultaneously avoiding toxic effects.

CANDIDATE RADIONUCLIDES

Many radionuclides are candidates for use in endovascular brachytherapy. Selected properties of some of these radionuclides are shown in Table 16-1.

The radioactive sources currently under investigation range in activity from a low of 20 kilobequerel (kBq) (0.5 μCi) to a high of 370 gigabequerel (GBq) (10 Ci). Very few other areas of medicine involve a 10 million to 1 range for the treatment of the same entity. Sources with activities in the kilobequerel to megabequerel range are permanently implanted. They deliver their treatment at low dose rates (LDR). High-activity sources (gigabequerel) are placed in position for a few minutes. These treatments are administered at high dose rates (HDR).

TABLE 16-1. Possible radionuclides for endovascular brachytherapy

Nuclide	Emissions	Half-Life	Deployment
^{32}P	Beta	14.3 days	LDR stent or HDR removable
^{90}Y	Beta	64 hours	HDR removable
^{90}Sr/Y	Beta	28 years	HDR removable
^{99m}Tc	Beta and Photon	6 hours	Direct injection
^{103}Pd	Photon	17 days	LDR stent
^{133}Xe	Beta	5.2 days	HDR removable
^{192}Ir	Gamma	74 days	HDR removable

PRINCIPAL DELIVERY SYSTEMS

The three main delivery systems under consideration are LDR radioactive stents, HDR solid sources, and HDR gas- or liquid-filled balloons. Generic versions of these systems are discussed in this section.

Radioactive Stents (Low Dose Rate)

A typical radioactive stent is shown in Figure 16-1. Versions of this device are manufactured by implanting ^{32}P or ^{103}Pd onto the surface of a standard cardiac stent. It is also possible to activate certain stents with a cyclotron beam. These are durable processes. Little of the radionuclide will be shed from the device during normal handling or while it is in the patient.

The radioactive stent is permanently deployed at the site of the lesion. The treatment is given over a prolonged time as the radionuclide decays. One benefit of the extended treatment time is the very low required activity. At the time of this writing, almost all clinical experience has been obtained using ^{32}P, a beta emitter. Typical initial source strengths are in the range of 20–2000 kBq ($\approx$0.5–50 Ci). The dose rate declines over time. Three quarters of the total radiation dose is delivered in the month following implantation.

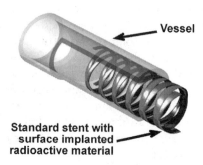

FIG. 16-1. Generic radioactive stent. A standard stent is prepared either by implanting radioactive ions or by making the stent's metal active.

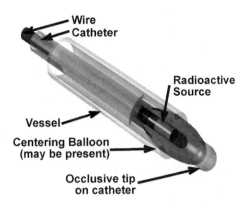

FIG. 16-2. Generic HDR solid source. In this example, a single solid source is mounted on the end of a delivery wire. Note that the occlusive catheter tip isolates the delivery system from the patient's blood.

There are substantial differences in biological response to LDR radiation compared with HDR treatments. This is due to tissue repair mechanisms, which are important whenever the treatment time exceeds an hour or so. The interaction between repair mechanisms and a treatment extended over many cell cycles is complex.

Removable Solid Sources (HDR)

A typical HDR solid source is shown in Figure 16-2. A wire is used to position the single source shown in this example. This construction is typical of the HDR devices used for cancer therapy in the past three decades. Some endovascular devices are quite similar to this conceptual model. Other available devices use a ribbon of multiple small sources at the end of the wire (Figs. 16-3 and 16-4). Other systems use individual small sources with hydraulic positioning means.

All forms of such devices isolate the delivery system from the patient's blood and provide means for rapid removal of the entire system from the patient when required. To minimize the likelihood of intimal injury, most

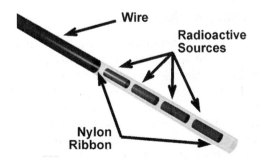

FIG. 16-3. HDR source assembly. A ribbon of small sources provides anatomic coverage while retaining flexibility.

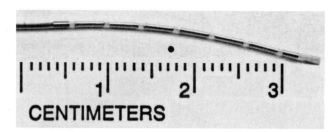

FIG. 16-4. Photograph of a source ribbon. The delivery wire is to the left. Six sources are present. Small markers proceed and follow the active sources. The dot above the scale represents a typical prescription point.

catheter designs maintain an appropriate minimum spacing between the source and the arterial wall.

Treatment time can be calculated once the prescription point and the type of the radionuclide are known. Typical treatment times range from a few minutes using 1 GBq of ^{90}Sr/^{90}Y to a few tens of minutes using 10 GBq of ^{192}Ir. A radiation therapy HDR treatment is administered over a few minutes by robotically moving a single 300 GBq ^{192}Ir source in a preplanned sequence.

For any given radionuclide, increasing the activity of the source decreases the treatment time. The need to deploy the source in a small vessel constrains its physical size of the treatment capsule. The maximum activity of most of the radionuclides shown in Table 16-1, which can be inserted into a clinically usable capsule, is much higher than that needed to meet clinical requirements.

Too long a treatment time is undesirable because of the increased risk of leaving the catheter across the lesion for a prolonged interval. Too short a treatment time may not allow adequate time to react to clinical requirements such as precisely positioning the source train.

As a source is deployed, it will irradiate tissue along its path. Hot sources increase the degree of this unwanted irradiation. There may also be a substantial distance between the shielded source container and the entry point of the catheter into the patient. Decreasing deployment time lowers staff transit dose. Increasing deployment time lowers the probability of displacing the catheter or of a mechanical complication.

Removable Fluid Sources (HDR)

A typical fluid-filled balloon system is shown in Figure 16-5. A balloon is positioned in the lesion and inflated with a radioactive liquid or gas. Diseased arterial lumens are seldom concentric and circular in cross section. Fully expanded balloons tend to self-center in the available lumen. When filled with a radioactive fluid, this arrangement delivers a reasonably uniform dose to the surface of lumen. Because of nonuniform residual plaque, the dose distribution to target tissues is likely to be nonuniform.

This technology, however, also has its challenges. Balloons might leak or, on very rare occasions, burst and spill their contents into the patient's bloodstream. Extensive sets of contingency plans are required. The radioactive ma-

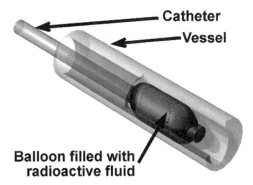

FIG. 16-5. Generic HDR fluid source. The balloon is expanded using a radioactive fluid. This may provide a more uniform dose to the arterial wall.

terials need to be physiologically cleared from the patient before an unacceptable dose is delivered to any tissue. Spills of radioactive liquids outside the patient have already occurred. The resultant radioactive contamination of the laboratory usually requires closure of the facility for several days.

SOURCE DELIVERY

A generic in-laboratory transfer system is shown in Figure 16-6. The source containers for both beta and gamma sources are designed to reduce the dose rate on their surfaces to an acceptable level. High-energy X-ray production (bremsstrahlung) by beta sources inside a container is a contributor to surface dose. One should avoid standing near or handling a loaded container.

To avoid mechanical transfer problems, the system should be aligned so that there are no sharp curves in the treatment catheter between the container and the patient's entry sheath. It is prudent to verify a clear channel by inserting an inactive wire (often called a dummy source) before deploying the active source. Both of these principles are standard practice in HDR cancer

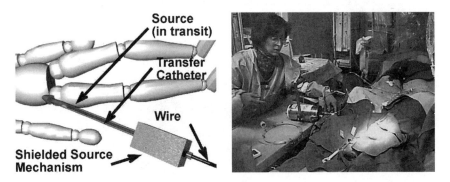

FIG. 16-6. Source delivery. The radiation oncologist is shown hooking up the system prior to treatment.

therapy. They have been adapted to endovascular brachytherapy (EVBT) systems.

CLINICAL DOSIMETRY

Anatomic Considerations

An absolute requirement for all forms of radiation therapy is that therapeutic dose must be delivered to the target tissue without exceeding a toxic dose to any other tissue. As of this writing, the EVBT target is assumed to be the arterial adventitia. Prescription doses from the different protocols deliver an adventitial dose ranging from 5 to 20 Gy.

Patient anatomy is seldom as geometrically symmetric as is often portrayed in physics textbooks (Figs. 16-7 and 16-8). For both ideal and real anatomy, the treatment system needs to have dosimetric characteristics suitable for delivery of an appropriate therapeutic dose to the target tissue without overdosing the intima.

In the ideal situation (Fig. 16-7), the dose delivered to the prescription point is determined by the source geometry, the anatomy of the artery, and the radial dose function of the selected radionuclide. The effect of source geometry is minimized by centering the source in the lumen (and in the artery in this case). This minimizes the geometric difference in dose delivered to the intima vs. the target.

Radiation Fields Around a Brachytherapy Source

The radiation field close to a point brachytherapy source is nonuniform. The radiation flux at any particular point in tissue is determined by four major factors. These are the intensity of the source, the inverse-square law, the absorption of radiation, and the scatter of radiation. The half-life of the source radionuclide is an additional consideration for permanent implants.

Consider a hypothetical source that emits radiation that is neither attenuated nor scattered. The relative distribution of radiation around such a source is defined only by geometrical factors.

Figure 16-9 illustrates three equal activity sources of radiation. For discussion purposes, we assume that each source is a mathematical point and that

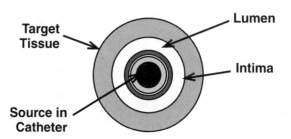

FIG. 16-7. Ideal treatment geometry. The source is centered in the lumen and the lumen is centered in the artery. This only occurs in physics textbooks.

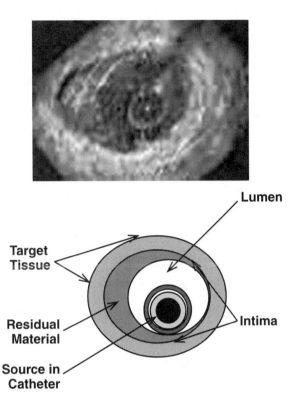

FIG. 16-8. Typical treatment geometry. The source is not centered in the eccentric lumen and the lumen is not centered in the eccentric artery. The treatment system is expected to deliver an appropriate therapeutic dose without injuring the intima.

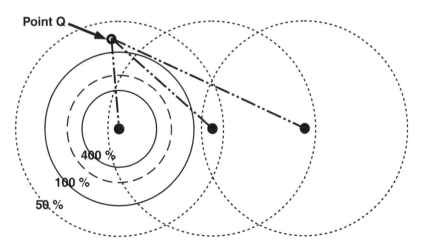

FIG. 16-9. Isodose curves surrounding three point sources of radiation. The dose at point Q includes contributions from all three sources.

the inverse square law is the only factor affecting the radiation distribution. The isodose surfaces are spheres. The intersection of the left 50% isodose sphere with the plane of Figure 16-9 gives a 50% isodose circle. Some additional isodose lines are also shown for the left source.

The total dose at a point such as Q is obtained by adding the contributions made by each source. If needed, the calculations can be refined using such factors as source asymmetry, tissue attenuation, and scatter.

Figure 16-10 shows the isodose curves calculated for 1, 3, 7, and 13 source ribbons. These computations were made using commercial software used in conjunction with a HDR remote afterloader intended for cancer treatments.

Figure 16-11 illustrates the relationship between the location of the prescription point and the number of sources making a substantial contribution to the dose at that point. As shown in the inserted scale drawing, prescription points ranging from 1 to 4 mm above the axis are centered above the line of sources.

Fewer sources contribute substantial dose to the prescription point when it is close to the line. As an example, consider five active sources: The dose delivered to increasingly remote prescription points is a decreasing fraction (i.e., 95, 87, 81, 76%) of the full ribbon dose at the same points.

Nonuniform Source Loading

Restenosis at the ends of the treated volume is a real concern. (The treated volume needs to cover the entire area traumatized by the intervention plus adequate margins.) Hot end treatments can extend the treatment zone further along the artery. The "cost" is increased intimal dose. Sets of isodose curves

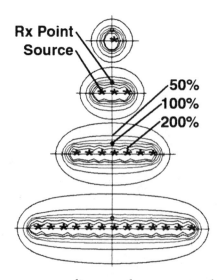

FIG. 16-10. Isodose curves surrounding one, three, seven, and thirteen sources. The 200%, 150%, 100%, 75%, 50%, and 25% isodose lines are shown. All doses are relative to 100% at the prescription point. The commercial treatment planning software normalized the dose to 100% at the prescription point (2 mm above the line of sources).

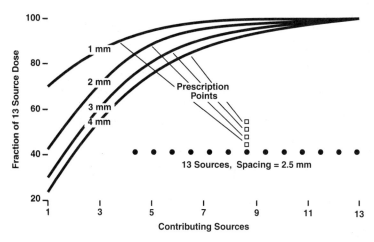

FIG. **16-11.** **Effective sources.** The closer the prescription point is to a line of sources, the fewer the number of sources that make a substantial contribution to the dose at that point.

from a 13-source string are shown in Figure 16-12. All four plans have been normalized to deliver 100% at 2 mm above the central source.

Plan A represents the equal strength model discussed in the previous paragraphs. The three-dimensional isodose distribution is a cylinder with rounded ends. The length of this cylinder is determined by the length of the source string. End restenosis might be minimized by using a source string that extends well beyond the ends of the angioplasty region.

Plan B pushes the 100% isodose line away from the ends of the ribbon by increasing the strength of each end source by a factor of four. *Plan C* increases

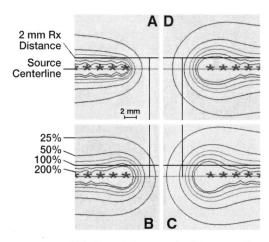

FIG. **16-12.** **Isodose curves with differential source loading.** A: All sources in the ribbon have the same strength. B: One source at the end has 4 times the strength of the others. (High-dose region extended.) C: One end source is 8 times. (High-dose region extends radially.) D: The two end sources are each 4 times. (High-dose region extends along the artery.)

the strength of each end source by a factor of eight. *Plan D* increases the strength of the two sources at each end of the string by a factor of four. Note the radial extension of the high dose region in *plans B, C,* and *D*.

The "dumbbell"-shaped isodose distributions produced by nonuniform source loading are well known in cancer therapy. Dumbbell loaded radium needles were used a half century ago. These needles were inserted into tumors. Overkill of small volumes of a cancer is not a problem.

The need to avoid delivering a toxic dose to the intima limits the maximum allowable differential loading. As previously discussed, the dose to the prescription point is delivered by the central sources. The dose to the intima is delivered by the closest source. Hot ends increase the intimal dose at the ends of the source train without substantially affecting the dose to the prescription point.

DIFFERENT RADIONUCLIDES

Physical Dose Distribution

The central dose-delivery problem in vascular brachytherapy is that the source is inside the artery, whereas the target tissue is outside the artery. Therefore, for geometric reasons alone, the intima will always receive a higher dose than the target.

Biological effects are caused by the interaction of high-energy electrons with tissue. In the case of a beta source, the beta particles are themselves the electrons. In the case of a gamma source, primary interactions of the gamma rays with tissue produce high-energy electrons in situ. Thus, beta and gamma sources can be considered two delivery mechanisms for the same active agent.

High-energy electrons, from any source, dissipate their energy after they pass through a short distance in tissue. This distance is determined by the initial electron energy. Adjustable energy electron accelerators are in common use for radiation oncology. Penetration depth in tissue is controlled by selecting an appropriate energy.

High-energy photons are exponentially attenuated by tissue. The half-value layer for ^{192}Ir gamma rays is several centimeters. Thus, there is minimal attenuation of the photon intensity over the few millimeters of importance to vascular brachytherapy. However, the electrons produced by photon interactions with tissue dissipate their energy within less than a millimeter of the interaction point.

The dose at any point has contributions from all of the electrons within range of that point. This includes contributions from electrons scattered from elsewhere in the tissue.

The effects of attenuation and scatter may be described by a radial dose function (RDF). The RDF is defined in such a way that geometric effects (i.e., the inverse square law) and mechanical considerations (i.e., physical design of the source) are excluded. Figure 16-13 shows the RDF for ^{90}Sr/Y. The horizontal dotted line depicts the result when the effects of scatter and attenuation are neglected. This line is also the approximate RDF for ^{192}Ir. For teaching

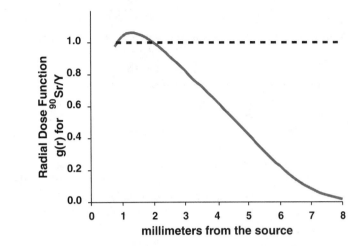

FIG. 16-13. Radial dose function for ^{90}Sr/Y. The radial dose function displays the effects of attenuation and scatter on the intensity at a distance from the source. The effect of the inverse square law has been removed. The dotted line is the approximate RDF for ^{192}Ir. [Adapted from Soares (1999)]

purposes, the following discussion concentrates on these two widely used EVBT radionuclides. To avoid mathematical complexity, the ideal geometry shown in Figure 16-7 is also assumed to be valid.

The RDF for ^{90}Sr/Y is higher than 1.0 for distances less than 2 mm from the source. This is because backscatter from deeper in the tissue contributes more to local dose than attenuation removes. The maximum range of beta particles produced by the ^{90}Sr/Y combination is less than 8 mm. The RDF falls essentially to zero at 8 mm.

The RDF for ^{192}Ir is approximately constant because there is little attenuation of the gamma photons over the 8 mm distance indicated in the figure. Thus, equal numbers of electrons are generated (and deliver their contribution to dose) at all points along the range.

The Choice of Radionuclide

The choice of radionuclide selection should be based on the radial dose function. In an ideal geometry, from a dosimetric point of view, the choice between ^{90}Sr/Y and ^{192}Ir depends on the arterial size and the maximum acceptable ratio between intimal and target doses.

There is no reason to select one radionuclide over the other if the prescription point is within 2 mm of the center of the artery. This is because the RDF for both radionuclides is essentially one at these distances.

The ^{90}Sr/Y system cannot be used if the prescription point is more than 8 mm from the source. This is because the beta particles cannot penetrate 8 mm of tissue.

Selecting a source is a complex issue at intermediate distances. Consider the ideal geometry shown in Figure 16-7. If the intima is at 2 mm and the target is at 4 mm, then the RDF for ^{90}Sr/Y is 68%. Delivery of equal target dose means that the intima receives 47% more dose when ^{90}Sr /Y is selected in place of ^{192}Ir. The importance of this increase turns out to depend on the maximum allowable intimal dose and the arterial wall thickness. There is some maximum arterial size appropriate for ^{90}Sr/Y treatments.

The choice is further complicated in real arteries (Figure 16-8). Here, one is faced with the necessity of delivering an adequate dose to the furthest target while protecting the closest portion of the intima. The practical effect is a reduction in the maximum vessel size for ^{90}Sr/Y.

The choice of other combinations of radionuclides and deployment systems are calculable using the basic principles described above. The ultimate decision will be based on better knowledge of the location of the target and of the radiation tolerance of the intima. Once the radiotherapeutic facts are known, one can refine the selection to include additional safety and operational efficacy factors.

RADIATION SAFETY

Both beta and gamma HDR sources deliver therapeutic doses of radiation in a matter of minutes. Direct contact of a physically small HDR source with tissue is hazardous. Brief contact can produce a major radiation burn.

Patient

The principal patient risk is the loss of control of a HDR source during treatment. The effect of such a loss can be catastrophic. Details of emergency planning, ongoing quality assurance, and operational procedures are specific to individual systems. However, some general guidelines for solid sources are given in the following paragraphs.

A medical event can be expected during a small fraction of the treatments. Potential causes include the patient's underlying condition, the occlusive effects of the treatment device, and drug reactions. When such an event occurs, the source should be withdrawn using normal techniques.

The source might be impeded or stopped during deployment or withdrawal. The best defense against such an occurrence is to using an inert wire to test the entire delivery channel into the patient immediately before source deployment. If the source "hangs-up" while it is in transit, a brief attempt should be made to withdraw it normally. The fallback position is to withdraw the treatment catheter and the source as a single unit. The catheter (containing the source) is then placed into an appropriate (lead for gamma, plastic for beta) emergency container. To avoid dropping the source in the lab, the catheter should not be cut or disconnected from the treatment device.

The source might become disconnected from its transport mechanism. (This has happened during a cancer HDR treatment with a single 300 GBq source.) Should this happen, the source is usually somewhere in the closed delivery system. End of treatment source-withdrawal must be verified both by system-specific mechanical means and by mandatory radiation measurements of the patient and treatment catheter. Here again, the fallback position is to withdraw the treatment catheter and place it in the emergency container.

There are some nonemergency patient-radiation safety concerns. Cancer induction is one such item. Indeed, the risk of a late cancer was one of the primary reasons for not using radiation therapy for the treatment of benign disease. The situation with regard to postradiation angioplasty is more complex. The interventional procedure itself requires a significant irradiation of the patient. The additional cancer risk from EVBT is a small fraction of the radiation risk from the angioplasty. Given that EVBT reduces restenosis and the need for complex reintervention, there may even be a net reduction in cancer risk.

Patients, their families, and general hospital staff may have concerns about residual radiation effects following EVBT. Questions are asked regarding the radiation hazard that a treated patient poses to others. Staff training, along with patient and family counseling, is essential for addressing unwarranted fears. There is no problem. The minute amount of ^{32}P used in radioactive stents is difficult to measure outside of the patient. Patients are not radioactive once a source is removed.

Staff

Beta particles are essentially absorbed by the patient's tissues or by a 1- to 2-cm-thick plastic shield. Staff exposure from a beta source deep in the patient is not significant. High-energy beta particles have a range of several meters in air.

Radiation is measurable for a distance of several meters around the patient being treated with a gamma source. This is more an expression of the sensitivity of radiation measuring instruments than an indication of a hazardous workplace.

Much of the remainder of this section deals with radiation protection from high-energy gamma sources. However, the radiation risk from exposed beta sources cannot be neglected.

The basic rules of radiation protection discussed in Chapter 14 still apply. The application of these rules for an iridium source is somewhat different because the half-value-layer in lead for ^{192}Ir gamma rays is much higher than the fluoroscopic value. Conventional fluoroscopic aprons offer virtually no protection from high-energy gamma photons. Fluoroscopic exposure rates outside the lead apron greatly exceed those produced by EVBT gamma sources. Lead aprons are necessary protection for fluoroscopic and fluorographic portions of the procedure.

A shielded bail-out box is placed in the laboratory to receive the source (and catheter) in the rare case of an emergency. This container is made of lead for a gamma source or plastic for a beta source.

Portable therapy shields are available for use with gamma sources. These may be required under certain circumstances such as small laboratories, special populations in adjacent spaces, and high procedure volumes. Regulatory limits define when the use of additional shielding is mandatory. It is good practice to always use available shields. Two forms of gamma shield are available. Small shields may be placed close to the patient (Fig. 16-14). This provides addi-

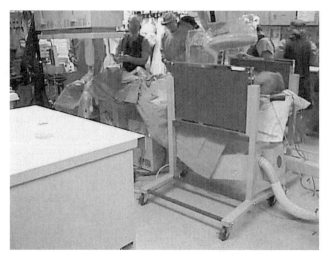

FIG. 16-14. Small shield. These 25-mm-thick lead shields will attenuate the ^{192}Ir gamma field behind them by more than 90%. [Photographed at the Scripps Institute, La Jolla, CA]

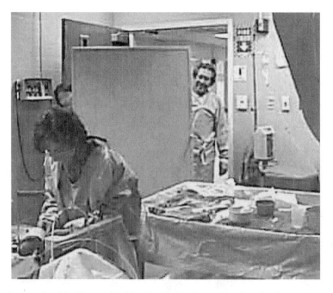

FIG. 16-15. Large shield. These shields are also 25 mm thick. The larger size provides an appropriate large shadow region behind the shield. This design improves patient access when the shield is far from the table. [Photographed at Lenox Hill Hospital, New York, NY]

tional protection for the radiation team. Large shields may be placed at a distance from the patient (Fig. 16-15). This provides normal access to the patient when necessary.

Distance and time play the major roles in reducing staff dose from both beta and gamma sources. Personnel monitoring experiments and records of personnel have shown that a single team can perform several hundred procedures per year without exceeding a small fraction of any individual's MPD.

Situational awareness is enhanced by keeping a radiation detector with an audible output on the treatment cart. The audible count rate provides feedback to the team about the source position. An unusual situation, such as failure to fully retract the source into the delivery device, is immediately apparent.

A posttreatment survey of the patient and laboratory eliminates the possibility of a lost source becoming a radiation hazard. Such a survey is easy if a gamma source is used for treatments. Sensitive instruments are able to detect the bremsstrahlung produced by most beta sources.

Disposal of Radioactive Materials

Table 16-2 gives the required radioactive decay times required before disposing of each of our candidate radionuclides. (The decay time for a mother-daughter pair, such as $^{90}Sr/^{90}Y$, is equal to that of the mother.) In Table 16-2, it is assumed that a 37-Bq (1 nCi) source can be considered nonradioactive. Long-lived radioactive devices that have ended their clinical utility must be disposed of by transfer to an authorized party.

Operational and Regulatory Considerations

Because the potential hazard is higher with therapy than that associated with diagnostic procedures, the corresponding degree of regulatory oversight is more intense. Most jurisdictions require a specific radionuclide license for each type of therapeutic procedure.

Resources are needed to safely manage radioactive material. Secure control of the radioactive inventory is of special concern. The administrative hazards and real dangers from misplaced radioactive materials cannot be overstated.

TABLE 16-2. Time required for a source to decay to 37 Bq (1 nCi)

Nuclide Half life	^{99m}Tc 6 hours	^{90}Y 2.7 days	^{133}Xe 5.2 days	^{32}P 14.3 days	^{103}Pd 17 days	^{192}Ir 74 days	^{90}Sr 28 years
Initial activity	Hours			Months			Years
370 GBq 930	10 Ci	8.3	3.0	5.8	15.8	18.8	6.7
370 MBq 651	10 mCi	5.8	2.1	4.0	11.1	13.2	4.7
370 kBq 372	10 μCi	3.3	1.2	2.3	6.3	7.5	2.7

MINI COURSE

Beta and gamma sources are essentially two different delivery mechanisms for the same drug (ionization-induced DNA damage).

Successful vascular brachytherapy requires the combined skills of a multidisciplinary team.

The use of therapeutic levels of radionuclides in the interventional laboratory calls for special safety precautions.

SECTION FIVE

Quality Assurance

17

Quality Assurance

THE QUALITY PROCESS

Quality assurance (QA) is often defined as "a system of procedures carried out to ensure that a product or a system adheres to established standards." This definition implies the existence of established standards as well as the compliance procedures. The elements of an operational QA program are testing and acting to maintain compliance.

Quality performance is obtained by purchasing systems that meet clinical needs, acceptance testing to ensure initial quality, and periodic testing. Items out of compliance are repaired to restore performance. The repairs are then tested. There is a myriad of tools and tests available for testing individual imaging components and for service purposes. Component level testing is too specific to each particular model of equipment to be covered generically.

The operator becomes part of the control loops in the imaging system. Appropriate quality images can only be achieved when operators understand how their actions affect imaging parameters and patient dose.

Quality = compliance with requirements. This may not be the best possible performance.

WHAT AND WHEN TO TEST?

The traditional test program for an imaging system was based on the measurement of individual components (e.g., focal-spot size) and indicator accuracy (e.g., kVp). This dates from a time when a hospital might assemble its own system using components purchased from different vendors and when most controls were open loop. Neither of these situations applies to current interventional fluoro systems.

Component and system level tests should be performed when a new system is installed. This establishes a performance baseline. Periodic component testing is seldom needed if system performance tests give acceptable results. Component testing is done to identify the cause of poor system performance.

System level tests should be routinely performed twice a year. Additional testing is needed for unstable systems or after major repairs. Individualized judgment, including attention to operators' comments regarding system performance, is important.

SPECIFICATION AND SIMULATION OF CLINICAL REQUIREMENTS

There is no sharp division between acceptable and unacceptable imaging performance. The ability of a physician to use an image is dependent on the technical quality of the image, prior information about the patient, the physician's experience, and other factors. There is a nonlinear relationship between the technical quality of an image and its medical utility. An operator only needs to see enough information in an image to confidently make necessary clinical decisions. Very poor images are usually unacceptable. Up to a point, improvements in technical image quality usually result in increased probability of medical utility. At some point, the image is good enough so that further increases in quality are unlikely to significantly increase the medical utility of the procedure. This level of performance is seldom near the upper limits of technically achievable image quality.

The definition of quality given at the start of this chapter includes the concept of conforming to established standards. Meeting this requirement does not mean that the absolute best image is required under all circumstances. Too good an image is wasteful. One must consider both the dollar and radiation costs of excess imaging performance. Micromanagement of dose and image quality is distracting. It is therefore prudent to set up systems with a bit more imaging performance and dose than the absolute minimum requirements.

The performance of any medical imaging system can be divided into two categories: suitability of the images for the clinical procedure (image quality factors) and the amount of energy administered to the patient while images are acquired (dose factors). Variability in clinical needs means that a performance threshold cannot be rigorously defined. It cannot be said that performance below any specified value never yields a useful image and performance at the same specified value is always useful. Nevertheless, performance thresholds appear in professional and regulatory documents. These are derived by "translating" the need to see clinical targets (e.g., fine vessels) into technically measurable tests (e.g., spatial resolution).

CHARACTERIZATION OF IMAGING PERFORMANCE

The performance of an imaging system can be characterized by methods ranging from subjective clinical opinion, through phantom testing with human interpretation of results, to analytic interpretation of digital test images. An example of a specific fluoroscopic system phantom is discussed later in this chapter. (Some of the material in this section requires familiarity with the tests built into this representative phantom.)

There are always observed variations in performance when the *same* phantom is used to test a series of imaging systems. A range of results is seen both for image quality parameters (e.g., spatial resolution) and for radiation (e.g., phantom entrance exposure rate). A histogram of the entrance exposure rate (EER) into the phantom for a large number of systems is sketched in Figure 17-1.

The extended tail in the high-rate region (solid columns in the drawing) is a typical finding. This tail is composed of systems with worn-out image intensifiers, improperly serviced systems, and instances of users routinely selecting too high a dose rate. Operating a system with dose rates in this region is usually unjustifiable in an interventional laboratory.

The few systems at the end of the tail deliver very high EERs. There is an increasing regulatory movement toward establishing "reference doses." Data are collected, and a histogram of EERs is obtained. The "reference dose" is typically set at the 75th percentile of the cumulative distribution. Systems operating above this level are investigated to determine the reason for high dose. Servicing the system can usually reduce EERs to a more acceptable level. Note that applying this process repeatedly could result in inappropriate performance. At some point in time, absolute procedure-specific reference doses will be needed.

Systems with too low an EER should also be investigated (hatched column in Fig. 17-1). A cross-check is made against imaging performance (e.g., low-contrast detectability). Systems with low EER and excellent imaging performance are preferred. This is not always possible. Poor imaging performance might simply be attributable to an inadequate amount of radiation.

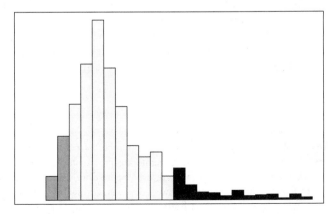

FIG. 17-1. EER histogram. Results from many systems tested with the same phantom. Too high an EER is poor practice. Too low an EER may be the cause of poor image quality.

A different result is obtained when EER is measured for a series of patients examined on the same system. The result is typically a normal distribution. Variability is due to patient variation. A typical distribution is illustrated in Figure 17-2a. For the purposes of this illustration, it was assumed that the imaging system was in good condition and that there were no limits on EER.

Regulatory limits exist. Systems are not allowed to exceed 10 R/min (under FDA test conditions). All of the heavy patients are now included in the last column of the histogram shown in Figure 17-2b. Images of these patients may have reduced image quality because of the dose limit.

The effects of limiting EER to 9 R/min are illustrated in Figure 17-2b. This may be due to a worn-out X-ray tube, excessive filtration, or an overly conservative service setting. In this figure, a large number of patients are examined using the limiting dose rate. Image quality for these patients might be reduced.

Automatic dose rate controls adjust X-ray output to match the patient from small patients up until technical or regulatory limits are encountered. This means that the limits have no effect on the dose delivered to small- or medium-sized patients.

It is desirable to displace the entire histogram to lower dose levels (Fig. 17-2d), provided that appropriate image quality is maintained. This ensures that appropriate examination of the widest possible range of patients has occurred.

A distribution of the maximum spatial resolution for a large number of the same model system measured with the same phantom is shown in Figure 17-3. The best achievable spatial resolution is determined by the system's design (right most column). Factors include the focal spot, the image intensifier, and the digital matrix size. Deterioration of the X-ray tube or image intensifier can only reduce spatial resolution (cross-hatched region).

The distribution of maximum spatial resolution over a number of makes and models of imaging systems will not have as sharp a maximum as that shown in the figure. The shallower decent is due to different optimizations made by different designers.

As mentioned above, the relationship between EER and low-contrast detectability (LCD) is more complex. Figure 17-4 shows histograms collected in a survey. EER may be either high or low, and LCD may be either better or worse (Table 17-1). One needs to simultaneously understand the location of the system under evaluation relative to both histograms in this figure.

FIG. 17-2. EER observed when a large number of patients are examined using the same system. **a: No dose limits.** All patients are presumably examined with appropriate image quality. Some receive high skin dose. **b: Some dose limits.** A few heavy patients are examined using the maximum allowed dose. Image quality might be adversely affected for these patients. **c: More dose limits.** A larger fraction of patients might be examined with diminished image quality. **d: A more sensitive system.** This may or may not adversely affect image quality. The very low dose region is of concern.

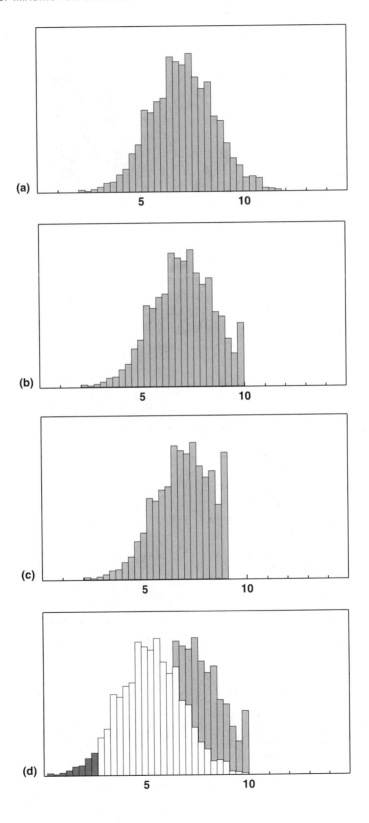

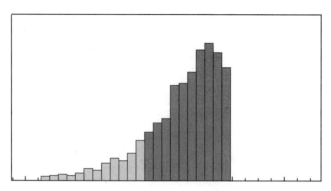

FIG. 17-3. Spatial resolution of a large number of the same model systems tested with the same phantom.

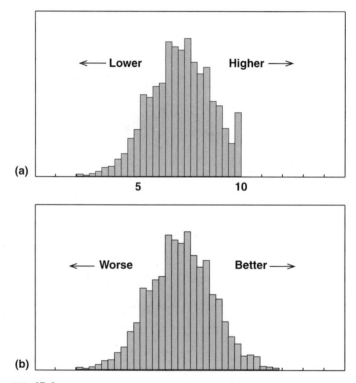

FIG. 17-4. a: Dose histogram. b: Low-contrast detectability histogram.

TABLE 17-1. Dose vs. low-contrast detectability

	Worse performance	Better performance
Low dose	Expected	Unusually good
High dose	Inadequate	Expected

CLINICAL REQUIREMENTS AND PERFORMANCE TESTS

Measurable differences in imaging test performance may or may not reflect meaningful differences in clinical utility. Uncertainties include the variety of clinical tasks for which the equipment might be used, differences in the skills of operators, and the lack of congruence between the phantom and patient tissue.

Patient entrance dose is only of value to the degree that it can predict the radiogenic risk of an examination. Patient entrance dose gives a qualitative estimate of risk. A precise calculation of risk requires knowledge of the X-ray spectrum, the distribution of dose within the patient, the distribution of tissues within the patient, the risk coefficients for individual tissues, and other factors.

Optimization requires a balance between the economic and medical benefits of an X-ray examination and the consequent economic cost and radiation risk. This balance is made either for an individual patient or for the group of patients that might be examined with the X-ray equipment under consideration. Among other factors, such calculations should include the economic value of human life; *the economic, medical, and social costs of not performing the procedure*; and the prevalence and severity of disease.

MEASUREMENT ACCURACY

The precision of an imaging measurement is affected by the observer. Decisions have to be made regarding the visibility of the lines and spaces in a bar pattern or the presence of a low-contrast target. Such decisions can be difficult. For example, most readers are familiar with the "which image is better" question during eyeglass fitting.

The problem is compounded when the observer is familiar with the phantom. It is not hard to identify targets when one knows where they are located. Random target locations provide more reliable performance data at the expense of increased measurement time and complexity.

An example of a randomized test is the measurement of low-contrast detectability by the four alternative forced choice method. In this test, a low-contrast target is randomly placed in one of four quadrants in a phantom. The observer must announce the quadrant containing the target. The test is passed if the observer successfully identifies the correct location in 9 of 12 trials.

Figure 17-5 illustrates this process. The target location is obvious in a, reasonably visible in b, and almost impossible to see in c. Other "random" phantoms are available.

NEMA FLUORO PHANTOM

It is worthwhile to examine the newly developed NEMA fluoro phantom in some detail. This phantom set was developed by a joint working group of the Society for Cardiac Angiography and Interventions and the National Electrical Manufacturers' Association (NEMA).

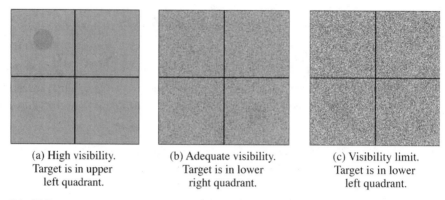

(a) High visibility. Target is in upper left quadrant.

(b) Adequate visibility. Target is in lower right quadrant.

(c) Visibility limit. Target is in lower left quadrant.

FIG. 17-5. Examples of four-alternative-forced-choice targets. a: High visibility. Target is in upper left quadrant. b: Adequate visibility. Target is in lower right quadrant. c: Visibility limit. Target is in lower left quadrant.

The system level tools described below are used to screen for inappropriate performance. Such tools are not always helpful in diagnosing the causes of such behavior. Supplementary tools can provide additional information about system or subsystem behavior. Equipment manufacturers recommend tools and procedures specific to the imaging systems that they supply.

A photograph of the phantom is shown in Figure 17-6. The center of the phantom is at the isocenter of the imaging system. Different thickness simulates a range of patient sizes and beam orientations.

The body of the phantom is constructed of polymethyl methacrylate (PMMA). This material has X-ray absorption and scattering properties similar to soft tissue. Thus, a stack of PMMA placed in the beam will drive the X-ray generator to an output level similar to that demanded by approximately the same tissue thickness.

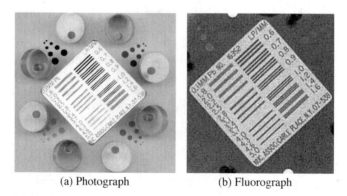

(a) Photograph

(b) Fluorograph

FIG. 17-6. Central portion of the NEMA phantom. The high- and low-contrast targets are seen. Note the discreet bar patterns in the high-contrast target. Portions of the working-thickness-range target are also seen. Also note the challenge targets overlying the air and aluminum cylinders.

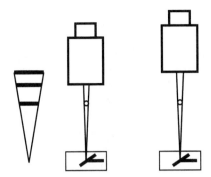

FIG. 17-7. Isocentric geometry. Organs of interest in a large patient are usually more magnified than in a small patient. It is assumed that the organ of interest is at the isocenter and that the image receptor is as close to the patient as practicable.

Test objects are positioned at the center of the phantom This simulates the location of clinically important organs. The phantom is usually positioned with its center at the X-ray system's isocenter. The image receptor is placed 5 cm above the top of the phantom. This simulates clinical imaging geometry. The geometric magnification of the test objects is similar to that of the clinical target (Fig. 17-7). Thus, receptor blur and focal spot penumbra blur are similar in test and clinical conditions.

X-ray scatter is also similar in both cases. Note that the entrance surface of a thick phantom is closer to the X-ray tube than the entrance surface of a thin phantom (Fig. 17-8). This is an additional reason why patient (phantom) dose increases with phantom thickness.

High-Contrast Resolution (Spatial Resolution)

High-contrast resolution is tested using a bar pattern (Table 17-2). The limiting resolution is determined by identifying the highest spatial frequency pattern in which 75% of the bars and spaces are identifiable. Discreet bars patterns were selected to minimize observation error.

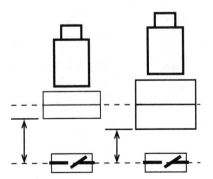

FIG. 17-8. Geometry. The SID increases and the SSD decreases as the phantom size increases (for a conventional angiographic system).

The bar pattern has a greater geometric magnification when centered in a thick phantom than when it is in a thin phantom. Systems with poor image-receptor resolution will have better spatial resolution when tested with thick phantoms. The increased magnification decreases the influence of the image receptor. Systems with oversized focal spots will have worse resolution when tested with thick phantoms because penumbra blur increases with magnification.

The limiting resolution of a conventional image intensifier increases as one zooms from a larger to a smaller field–of–view. The measured resolution is expected to increase as the field–of–view decreases.

When testing spatial resolution, the test plate is placed with the bars at 45° to the video lines or digital image matrix. This produces the smallest change in the Moiré pattern resulting from a small change in angle. Figure 17-9 illustrates the change from 0° to 2° as well as the 45° appearance.

Low-Contrast Detectability

Iodine detectability is tested by an array of iodine-epoxy cylinders of different diameters, depths, and iodine concentrations. Iodine detectability will increase as the phantom thickness decreases because the same iodine target produces greater subject contrast when imaged through a thin layer of plastic.

Motion Unsharpness

Motion unsharpness, camera lag, and the effects of recursive filtering are tested with a rotating spoke target. The spokes are angiographic–guide wires of different diameters. Two lead shot provide targets for evaluating the effects of camera lag and recursive filtering. The rotating wheel is also placed in the center of the phantom. Its drive motor is located outside of the field–of–view (Fig. 17-10).

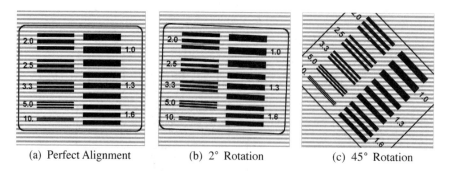

(a) Perfect Alignment   (b) 2° Rotation   (c) 45° Rotation

FIG. 17-9. Angular misalignment. Small angular misalignments make it difficult to interpret the bar pattern. Rotating the phantom 45° relative to the scan lines (or digital matrix) provide readings that are more consistent (see Fig. 17-6b). a: Perfect alignment. b: 2° rotation. c: 45° rotation.

TABLE 17-2. Relationship between object size and spatial resolution

Width of bar or space (mm)	Line pairs per millimeter
1.0	0.5
0.5	1.0
0.25	2.0
0.1	5.0
0.05	10.0

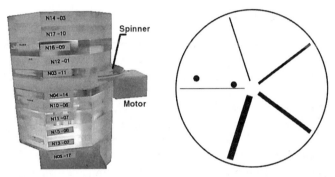

FIG. 17-10. Motion target. Positioned in the center of the phantom. The target wheel carries five guide wires and two lead shot. Note that the motor is outside of the phantom.

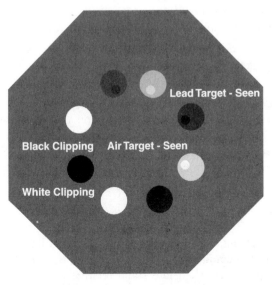

FIG. 17-11. Working thickness range. This sketch illustrates two examples of white clipping and one example of black clipping.

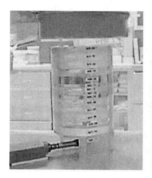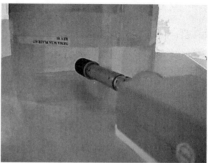

FIG. 17-12. Measurement of phantom entrance dose.

Working Thickness Range

Working thickness range is the ability to image structures overlaid by bone or air (Fig. 17-11). Systems with inadequate single-image latitude are unable to do this in bright (air) or dark (bone) portions of the image. The NEMA phantom contains eight cylinders composed of different heights of air, aluminum, and plastic. These cylinders are calibrated for a total 20-cm phantom thickness. A 25-mm-deep air challenge target overlaps the four air cylinders. The bright-side dynamic range is determined by how many of these targets are seen. A 5-mm lead challenge target overlaps the four aluminum cylinders. The dark-side dynamic range is determined by counting these targets.

Dosimetry

Phantom entrance dose is tested by placing an appropriate dosimeter at a fixed distance from the entrance surface of the phantom (Fig. 17-12). The systematic errors of a smaller distance to the focal spot and reduced scatter from the phantom partially offset each other. The results are acceptable for routine use.

HUMAN OR COMPUTER OBSERVERS?

Image quality test procedures are based on trained human observers. The consistency of these tests is dependent on the skill and training of the observer. The best approach to this is to enroll the testers in a formal training program before allowing them to work independently. The FDA has reached a similar conclusion in conjunction with their mammography regulations (MQSA).

UTILIZATION

The first use of this phantom will be the collection of dose and performance histograms similar to those shown in this chapter. Participants will benefit from knowing where their labs stand relative to the evolving database. Over time, correlations between measurements and subjective clinical impressions may provide the basis for reasonable performance benchmarks.

References

Attix, Frank, H. *Introduction to Radiological Physics and Radiation Dosimetry*. John Wiley and Sons (1986).

Bevelacqua, Joseph, J. *Basic Health Physics: Problems and Solutions*. John Wiley and Sons (1999).

Bushberg, Jerrold T. *The Essential Physics of Medical Imaging* (2nd ed.). Williams and Wilkins (1999).

Bushong, Stewart C. *Radiologic Science for Technologists: Physics, Biology, and Protection*. Mosby Year Book (1997).

Curry, Thomas S. III, Dowdey, James, E., and Murry, Robert C. *Christensen's Physics of Diagnostic Radiology*. Williams and Wilkins (1990).

Dowd, Steven B., and Tilson, Elwin R. *Practical Radiation Protection and Applied Radiobiology*. Harcourt Brace & Co. (1999).

Farr, R. F., and Allisy-Roberts, P. J. *Physics for Medical Imaging*. Saunders (1996).

Glagov S, Weisenberg E, Zarins CK, Stankunavicius R, Kolettis GJ. Compensatory enlargement of human atherosclerotic coronary arteries. *N Engl J Med* 1987;316(22):1371–5.

Haliday, D., Resnick R., and Kranek, J. *Physics* (4th ed.). New York: Wiley (1992).

Hall, Donald J. *Radiobiology for the Radiologist* (4th ed.). Lippincott-Raven Publishers (1993).

Holmes, D. R., Jr., Wondrow, M. A., Bell, M. R., et al. Cine Film Replacement: digital archival requirements and remaining obstacles. *Cath Cardiovasc Diagn* 44: 346–356, 1998.

International Commission on Radiological Protection. *The biological basis for dose limitation in the skin*. ICRP Publication 59. Ann ICRP 1991;22(2).

Johns, H. E., and Cunningham J. R. *The Physics of Radiology* (4th ed.). Springfield, IL: Charles C Thomas (1983).

Kassabian, M. K. *Roentgen Rays and Electro-Therapeutics with Chapters on Radium and Phototherapy* (2nd ed.). Philadelphia, PA: J B. Lippincott (1910). [Figure 209 A, Fig. 12-9.]

Kennedy, T. E., Nissen, S. E., Simon, R., Thomas, J. D., and Tilkemeier, P. L. *Digital Cardiac Imaging in the 21th Century: A Primer*. Cardiac and Vascular Information Working Group. Bethesda, MD: American College of Cardiology (1997).

Lichtenstein, D. A., Klapholz, L., Vardy, D. A., Leichter, I., Mosseri, M., Klaus, S. N., and Gilead, L. T. Chronic radiation dermatitis following cardiac catheterization. *Arch Dermatol* 132:663–667, 1996. [Fig. 12-1.]

Mettler, F. A., and Upton A. C. *Medical Effects of Ionizing Radiation* (2nd ed.). Philadelphia, PA: WB Saunders (1995).

Nelson, M., and Gailly, J. L. *The Data Compression Book.* IDG Books Worldwide (1995).

Perez, C., and Brady, L. *Principles and Practice of Radiation Oncology* (3rd ed.). New York: Lippincott-Raven Publishers (1997).

Rabbani, M., and Jones P. W. *Digital Image Compression Techniques.* Bellingham, WA: Society of Photo-optical Instrumentation Engineers (1991).

Rabbani, M., and Jones, P. W. Image compression techniques for medical diagnostic imaging systems. *J Digital Imag* 4:65–78 (1991).

Reiber, J. H. C., and Serruys, P. W. (Eds.) *Progress in Quantitative Coronary Arteriography.* Dordrecht: Kluwer Academic Publishers, p. 33–48 (1994).

Reiber, J. H. C., van der Wall, E. E. (Eds.) *What's New in Cardiovascular Imaging.* Dordrecht: Kluwer Academic Publishers, p. 31–46 (1998).

Schomer, D. F., Elekes, A. A., Hazle, J. D., et al. Introduction to wavelet-based compression of medical images. *RadioGraphics* 18:469–481, 1998.

Selman, Joseph. *Fundamentals of X-ray and Radium Physics* (8th ed.). Charles C. Thomas (1994).

Shope, T. B. Radiation-induced skin injuries from fluoroscopy. *RadioGraphics* 16:1195–1199, 1996. [Fig. 12-6].

Spralls, Perry, Jr. *Physical Principles of Medical Imaging.* Medical Physics Publishing. (1995).

Stone, M. S., Robson, K. J., and LeBoit, P. E. Subacute radiation dermatitis from fluoroscopy during coronary artery stenting: evidence for cytoxic lymphocyte mediated apoptosis. *J Am Acad Dermatol* 38:333–336, 1998 [Fig.12-2.]

Taylor, B. Guide for use of the international system of units (S). NIST Special Publication 811 (1995 edition). United States Government Printing Office, Washington DC, 1995.

Vañó, E., Arranz, L., Sastre, J. M., Moro, C., Ledo, A., Gárate, M. T., and Minguez, I. Dosimetric and radiation protection considerations based on some cases of patient skin injuries in interventional cardiology. *Brit J Radiol* 71:510, 1998 [Fig. 12-7.]

Vañó, E., Arranz, L., Sastre, J. M., Moro, C., Ledo, A., Gárate, M. T., and Minguez, I. Dosimetric and radiation protection considerations based on some cases of patient skin injuries in interventional cardiology. *Brit J Radiol* 71:510, 1998 [Fig. 12-8.]

Vañó, E., Gonzalez, L., Beneytez, F., and Moreno, F. Lens injuries induced by occupational exposure in non-optimized interventional radiology laboratories. *Brit J Radiol* 71:728–733, 1998 [Fig. 12-12.]

Wagner, L. K., and Archer, B. A. *Minimizing Risks from Fluoroscopic X Rays—Bioeffects, Instrumentation and Examination* (2nd ed.). Houston, TX: Partners in Radiation Management (1998). [Fig. 12-4.]

Wagner, L. K., and Archer, B. A. *Minimizing Risks From Fluoroscopic X-Rays* (2nd ed.). Houston, TX: R.M. Partnership (1998).

Wagner, L. K., McNeese, M. D., Marx, M. V., and Siegel, E. L. Severe skin reactions from interventional fluoroscopy: case report and review of literature. *Radiology* 213:773–776, 1999. [Fig. 12-3.]

Wagner, L. K., Eifel, P. J., and Geise, R. A. Potential biological effects following high x-ray dose interventional procedures. *JVIR* 5:71–84, 1994.

Wolff, D., and Heinrich, K. W. Strahlenschäden der Haut nach Herzkatheterdiagnostik und therapie: 2 Kasuistiken. *Hautnah derm* 5:450–452, 1993. [Fig. 12-5.]

APPENDICES

APPENDIX A

Mass Attenuation Coefficients

	Muscle		Air		Water		Polymethyl methacrylate	
Density, g/cm^3	1.050		0.00121		1.000		1.190	
Energy, keV	μ	μ_{en}	μ	μ_{en}	μ	μ_{en}	μ	μ_{en}
10	5.356	4.964	5.120	4.742	5.329	4.944	3.357	3.026
15	1.693	1.396	1.614	1.334	1.673	1.374	1.101	0.832
20	0.821	0.564	0.778	0.539	0.810	0.550	0.571	0.333
30	0.378	0.161	0.354	0.154	0.376	0.156	0.303	0.096
40	0.269	0.072	0.249	0.068	0.268	0.069	0.235	0.046
50	0.226	0.043	0.208	0.041	0.227	0.042	0.207	0.031
60	0.205	0.033	0.188	0.030	0.206	0.032	0.192	0.025
80	0.182	0.026	0.166	0.024	0.184	0.026	0.175	0.023
100	0.169	0.025	0.154	0.023	0.171	0.025	0.164	0.024
150	0.149	0.027	0.136	0.025	0.151	0.028	0.146	0.027

	Bone, cortical		Aluminum		Copper		Iodine	
Density, g/cm^3	1.920		2.699		8.960		4.930	
Energy, keV	μ	μ_{en}	μ	μ_{en}	μ	μ_{en}	μ	μ_{en}
10	28.510	26.800	26.230	25.430	215.900	148.400	162.600	154.800
15	9.032	8.388	7.955	7.487	74.050	57.880	55.120	52.080
20	4.001	3.601	3.441	3.094	33.790	27.880	25.430	23.630
30	1.331	1.070	1.128	0.878	10.920	9.349	8.561	7.622
33.2 (I)	Value just below iodine K absorption edge						6.553	5.744
	Value just above iodine K absorption edge						35.820	11.880
40	0.666	0.451	0.569	0.360	4.862	4.163	22.100	9.616
50	0.424	0.234	0.368	0.184	2.613	2.192	12.320	6.573
60	0.315	0.140	0.278	0.110	1.593	1.290	7.579	4.518
80	0.223	0.069	0.202	0.055	0.763	0.558	3.510	2.331
100	0.186	0.046	0.170	0.038	0.458	0.295	1.942	1.342
150	0.148	0.032	0.138	0.028	0.222	0.103	0.698	0.474

Energy, keV	Iron 7.874 μ	μ_{en}	Platinum 21.450 μ	μ_{en}	Lead 11.350 μ	μ_{en}	CsI 4.510 μ	μ_{en}
10	170.600	136.900	113.200	107.800	130.600	124.700	171.100	162.400
15	57.080	48.960	157.800	126.500	111.600	91.000	58.150	54.860
20	25.680	22.600	75.740	63.330	86.360	68.990	26.860	24.960
30	8.176	7.251	26.410	22.680	30.320	25.360	9.045	8.071
33.2 (I)	Value just below iodine K absorption edge						6.923	6.088
	Value just above iodine K absorption edge						21.220	9.086
36.0 (Cs)	Value just below cesium K absorption edge						17.190	7.990
	Value just above cesium K absorption edge						30.270	10.590
40	3.629	3.155	12.450	10.670	14.360	12.110	22.970	9.395
50	1.958	1.638	6.954	5.879	8.041	6.740	12.870	6.596
60	1.205	0.956	4.339	3.595	5.021	4.149	7.921	4.586
78.4 (Pt)			2.203	1.738				
			9.301	2.627				
80	0.595	0.410	8.731	2.592	2.419	1.916	3.677	2.399
88 (Pb)					1.910	1.482		
					7.683	2.160		
100	0.372	0.218	4.993	2.081	5.549	1.976	2.035	1.391
150	0.196	0.080	1.795	1.006	2.014	1.056	0.729	0.495

APPENDIX B

International System (SI) of Units

SI prefixes

Multiplier	Name	Symbol	Multiplier	Name	Symbol
10^{-1}	deci	D	10^{1}	deka	da
10^{-2}	centi	C	10^{2}	hecto	h
10^{-3}	milli	M	10^{3}	kilo	k
10^{-6}	micro	μ	10^{6}	mega	M
10^{-9}	nano	N	10^{9}	giga	G
10^{-12}	pico	P	10^{12}	tera	T
10^{-15}	femto	F	10^{15}	peta	P
10^{-18}	atto	A	10^{18}	exa	E
10^{-21}	zepto	Z	10^{21}	zetta	Z
10^{-24}	yocto	Y	10^{24}	yotta	Y

SI base units

	Base quantity	Name
length	meter	m
mass	kilogram	kg
time	second	s
electric current	ampere	A
thermodynamic temperature	kelvin	K
amount of substance	mole	mol
luminous intensity	candela	cd

SI-derived units with special names and symbols*

Derived quantity	Name	Symbol	Expression in terms of other SI units	Expression in terms of SI base units
Frequency	hertz	Hz	—	s^{-1}
Energy, work, quantity of heat	joule	J	$N \cdot m$	$m^2 \cdot kg \cdot s^{-2}$
Power, radiant flux	watt	W	J/s	$m^2 \cdot kg \cdot s^{-3}$
Activity (of a radionuclide)	becquerel	Bq	—	s^{-1}
Absorbed dose, specific energy (imparted), kerma	gray	Gy	J/kg	$m^2 \cdot s^{-2}$
Dose equivalent**	sievert	Sv	J/kg	$m^2 \cdot s^{-2}$

*Other quantities, called *derived quantities*, are defined in terms of the seven base quantities Certain SI derived units have been given special names and symbols. Relevant examples are shown in this table.

**Other quantities expressed in sieverts, are ambient dose equivalent, directional dose equivalent, personal dose equivalent, and organ equivalent dose.

APPENDIX C

SI and Historical Radiation Units

SI radiation units with special names and symbols

	SI-derived unit	
Derived quantity	Name	Symbol
Exposure (X and gamma rays)*	coulomb per kilogram	C/kg
Absorbed dose rate	gray per second	Gy/s

*Air kerma has become the practical unit of exposure instead of C/kg.

Obsolete radiation units

Quantity	Symbol	Relation to SI Unit
Activity (Curie)	Ci	$= 3.7 \times 10^{10}$ Bq
Exposure (Roentgen)	R	$= 0.877$ cGy air kerma
Dose	Rad	$= 1$ cGy
Dose Equivalent	rem	$= 1$ cSv*

*The quality factor used for this conversion is one for X-rays, gamma rays, and beta particles. The quality factors for heavy particles (e.g., neutrons) differ.

APPENDIX D

A Partial List of Organizations of Interest

BEIR: *Biological Effects of Ionizing Radiation,* A committee of the United States National Academy of Science, which issues periodic reports on radiation. *www.nas.edu/cls/brerhome.nsf*

CDRH: *Center for Devices and Radiological Health,* The division of the FDA responsible for medical devices and radiological health. *www.fda.gov/cdrh*

CRCPD: *Conference of Radiation Control Program Directors,* Primary membership is made up of individuals in state and local government who regulate the use of radiation sources. *www.crcpd.org*

DICOM: *DICOM is a committee, not an organization,* Link via *nema.org*

FDA: *Food and Drug Administration,* The division of the United States federal government responsible for public health and similar matters. *www.fda.gov*

IAEA: *International Atomic Energy Agency,* A United Nations agency providing central resources for nuclear activities. *www.iaea.org*

ICRP: *International Commission on Radiological Protection,* A free-standing commission charged with developing and promulgating basic information on radiation safety. *www.icrp.org*

ICRU: *International Commission on Radiation Units,* A freestanding commission charged with developing and promulgating basic information on radiological units and measurements. *www.icru.org*

IEC: *International Electrotechnical Commission,* *http://www.iec.ch/*

NCRP: *National Council on Radiation Protection and Units,* *www.ncrp.com*

NEMA: *National Electrical Manufacturer's Association,* *www.nema.org*

NRC (USNRC): *Nuclear Regulatory Commission,* *www.nrc.gov*

UNSCEAR: *United Nations Scientific Committee on the Effects of Atomic Radiation,* Limited information available via *www.un.org*

APPENDIX E

Glossary

Absorbed: Retains the energy carried by radiation.

Afterloader: A brachytherapy treatment device that is placed into the patient empty. The sources are loaded at a later time.

Analog-to-digital converter (ADC): A device that converts an analog signal (e.g., a voltage level) into a digital value.

Anode: The positive element of an electronic device such as an X-ray tube.

As low as reasonably achievable (ALARA): The operational philosophy of reducing environmental radiation dose where practicable.

Attenuation: Reduction of the intensity of a radiation beam by absorption or scatter.

Attenuation coefficient: A measure of the X-ray attenuation properties of matter.

Automatic brightness control (ABC): A feedback circuit in an X-ray system intended to maintain the same scene brightness over a wide range of patient thickness. This is usually accomplished by controlling the X-ray output of the system.

Background radiation: The radiation level present before a particular source is deployed. Oftentimes, the content indicates that the natural level of background radiation is intended.

Backscatter: Scatter emerging from the area in which the X-ray beam enters the patient.

Bail-out-box: An appropriately shielded container into which a brachytherapy device can be dumped in case of necessity.

Bandwidth (digital): The number of bits that can be processed in a second.

Beam hardening: Increase in the average energy of a polychromatic beam by preferentially absorbing lower energy photons.

Beam quality: Penetrating ability of an X-ray beam

Beta particles: High-energy electrons emitted by the nucleus of nuclei that contain too many or too few neutrons.

Bit depth: The number of bits of digital information available to describe the brightness of a pixel.

Brachytherapy: Radiation therapy delivered with short distances between the sources and target point.

Bremsstrahlung: X-ray photons formed when high-energy electrons are stopped by their interaction with matter. Literally, "braking radiation."

Bucky: A moving radiographic grid.

Cathode: Negative element of an electronic device such as an X-ray tube.

Cathode ray tube (CRT): A vacuum tube, such as a television monitor that uses electrons (cathode rays) to form the image.

Central ray: A mathematical line from the focal spot to the center of the X-ray beam.

Characteristic-fluorescent photon: Radiation with energies characteristic of the orbital electron levels of the absorbing atom.

Charged-coupled device (CCD): A solid-state device capable of forming a video signal from an optical image.

Cinefluorographic: Fluorographic recording at cine rates. This may be accomplished using either film or electronic means.

Client server: A computer network paradigm in which servers provide information to clients.

Closed loop: A control circuit incorporating feedback to regulate the observed signal.

Collimator: A device to constrain the size and shape of the X-ray beam.

Compton interaction: A photon loses a fraction of its energy to an atomic electron, A scattered secondary photon also emerges from the interaction.

Contrast: Difference in signal strength between a target and its background.

Contrast media: Material introduced into a structure to increase its radiographic contrast.

Controlled area: An area from which the public is excluded (for radiation protection purposes).

Conversion factor (G_x): A measure of the light produced by an image intensifier per unit of input X-ray dose.

Detector: A device that registers a response to a stimulus such as light or radiation.

Deterministic: A radiation effect having a dose threshold.

Diaphragm: A disk having a fixed or variable opening used to restrict the amount of light traversing a lens or optical system. An X-ray diaphragm similarly restricts an X-ray beam.

DICOM-CD: A combined logical and physical format intended to place cineangiograms onto a compact disk.

Digital subtraction angiogram (DSA): An angiograpic series comprised of a set of images from which a common "mask" image has been subtracted.

Digital-to-analog converter (DAC): Converts a digital number into an analog signal level (e.g., pixel brightness on a monitor).

Digitization: To put information into digital form.

Display: A device that gives information in visual form.

Display contrast: The portion of image contrast attributable to the characteristics and settings of the display device.

Dose: Energy absorbed at a "point" per unit mass. The "point" is the smallest volume in which the energy deposition is statistically uniform. This is substantially less than 1 mm^3 for diagnostic X rays in tissue.

Dose area product (DAP): Product of the entrance skin dose and the area of the X-ray beam at the entrance surface of the patient.

Dose equivalent (H): A quantity, defined for radiation protection purposes, that expresses on a common scale for all radiations, the irradiation incurred by exposed persons.

Dose rate: Dose delivered at a "point" per unit time.

Dosimeter: An instrument that measures the amount of radiation present at the measuring "point." In this case, the "point" is the size of the radiation detection element.

Dummy: An inert simulation of a radioactive device. Used to test the operation of the device and the eventual position of the active source.

Effective Dose(E): The sum over specified tissues of the products of the dose equivalent in a tissue and the weighting factor for that tissue.

Effective Dose Equivalent (H$_E$): The sum over specified tissues of the products of the dose equivalent in a tissue and the weighting factor for that tissue. Note: the weighting factors for E and H$_E$ differ.

Electromagnetic radiation: The propagation of a combined electric and magnetic field through space.

Electronic brightness gain: The degree of image-receptor gain attributable to electronic amplification.

Encoding: Conversion of a data element into a specific format.

Endovascular brachytherapy (EVBT): The application of radiation therapy to a vessel from within its lumen.

Entrance beam: The X-ray beam at the point where it enters the patient.

Exposure: A measure of the quantity of radiation present at a particular location. Exposure is formally determined by measuring air ionization.

Field of view (FOV): The maximum area that can be seen in an image.

Filament: The portion of the X-ray tube that is heated to produce electrons.

Film badge: A personal radiation monitor used to assess occupational exposure.

Film fluorography: Fluorography where the images are stored on film.

Film screen: An image receptor composed of film contained between radiographic intensifying screens.

Flicker: The perception of wavering light intensity caused by too low a repetition rate of the stimulus.

Fluorescence: The emission of light or characteristic X rays by the absorption of incident radiation and persisting only as long as the stimulating radiation is continued.

Fluorography: The digital or photographic record of x-ray images produced by a fluoroscope.

Fluoroscopy: The digital or photographic formation of non-recorded images.

ƒ Number: The ratio of the focal length of a lens or lens system to the effective diameter of its aperture. A lens with a small ƒ number is an efficient light collector.

Focal spot: The portion of the X-ray tube from which the useful beam originates.

Gamma rays: Photons emitted during nuclear de-excitation processes.

Geiger counter: An instrument that detects and measures radiation; consisting of a Geiger tube and associated electronics.

Granularity: Composed or appearing to be composed of grains.

Grid: A device to preferentially absorb scattered radiation rather than primary radiation.

Grid ratio: The ratio of the height of a grid strip divided by the space between two adjacent strips.

Half-life: The time necessary for one half of the nuclei in a sample of radioactive material to decay.

Half-value layer (HVL): The amount of attenuator needed to reduce the intensity of an X-ray beam by 50%.

Header: The portion of the logical contents of an X-ray image that describes both its own properties, the patient's demographics, and other relevant information.

Heat-storage capacity: The amount of energy that can be safely stored in a portion of an X-ray tube.

High dose rate (HDR): The delivery of brachytherapy treatments at dose rates exceeding 5 Gy/h at 1 cm from the source.

Hub: A computer network component capable of interconnecting several devices.

Image framing: The relationship between an image receptor field and the storage format. Overframed images neglect portions of the image receptor.

Image acquisition: Capturing and storing an image for latter use.

Image intensifier: An electro-optical device that converts an X-ray image into visible form. The brightness of the image is greater than that produced by a simple fluoroscopic screen.

Image receptor: A generic device for transuding an X-ray image into detectable form.

Image-noise: The noise content of an X-ray image.

Input phosphor: A layer of material at the entrance of an image receptor that emits fluorescent light when stimulated by X-rays.

Instant replay: The electronic replay of a fluorographic sequence immediately after acquisition.

Intensity: The strength of light or X-rays per unit area.

Interlaced scanning: A scheme in which the even and odd video scan lines are read or written as two separate fields.

International system of units (SI): An internationally accepted consistent set of physical units of measurement.

Inverse-square law: A mathematical description of the variation in intensity with distance from a point source

Ionization chamber: A radiation detector in which radiation produces measurable ionization events in a gas.

Isocenter: A mechanical location in a fluoroscopic system about which the major imaging components rotate. An object at isocenter remains in view as the gantry is rotated.

Isodose: A line or surface of constant dose.

Isokerma: A line or surface of constant kerma.

Justification: No practice involving exposure to radiation should be adopted unless it produces sufficient benefit to the exposed individuals to society to offset the radiation detriment it causes (ICRP).

K edge: A discontinuity on the attenuation coefficient that occurs at the binding energy of the K electrons of the attenuator.

Lag: The persistence of elements of a previous image in a later image.

Last-image hold: The process of recording and automatically replaying the last image of a fluoroscopic sequence.

Leakage radiation: Radiation emerging through the protective housing of an X-ray tube.

Line pairs per millimeter (lp/mm): A measure of spatial resolution. Higher values mean the ability to see smaller objects.

Linear attenuation coefficient: A measure of the X-ray attenuation properties per unit thickness of an attenuator.

Linear no threshold (LNT): A theory in which any amount of radiation caries a risk where the risk is proportional to dose.

Line-focus principle: An arrangement of the components of an X-ray tube so that the physical focus is larger than the effective focal spot.

Logical format: The formal organization of a set of digital data (e.g., a DICOM image).

Look-up table: A table defining the digital output value for a given input value.

Low contrast detectability (LCD): The ability to see an object that has small radiographic contrast relative to its background.

Low dose rate (LDR): The delivery of brachytherapy treatments at dose rates below the HDR limit.

Magnification: The projection of an image to a size larger than the original object.

Mass attenuation coefficient: A measure of the X-ray attenuation properties per unit mass of matter.

Maximum permissible dose (MPD): A regulatory limit for the amount of radiation that may be received by a person or organ.

Measuring field: An area in a radiographic scene from which the ABC feedback signal is derived.

Minification: The projection of an image to a size smaller than the original object.

Minification brightness gain: The degree of gain in an image-intensifier attributable to the reduction in area of the output screen relative to the input screen.

Modulation: The variation of the intensity of an X-ray beam caused by differential attenuation between an object and its surroundings.

Modulation transfer function (MTF): A graphical representation of the ability of an imaging device to reproduce objects of different sizes.

Monochromatic: A beam containing photons all with the same energy level (color).

Mother-daughter: The relationship between two radionuclides in a decay series.

Motion unsharpness: Image blur caused by motion of the object or imaging system.

Noise: A random disturbance that reduces the clarity of a signal.

Noncontrolled area: An area that the public might occupy (for radiation protection purposes).

Object-to-image-receptor Distance (OID): Distance between the object of interest and the entrance surface of the image receptor.

Occupational exposure: The amount of radiation encountered during one's occupation as a radiation worker.

Off-focus: Production of radiation in an X-ray tube outside of the defined focal spot.

Open loop: Control of a circuit without automatic feedback to regulate the level.

Optical density (OD): A logarithmic measure of the attenuation of light by a layer of film.

Optimization: Doses should be kept as low as reasonably achievable, economic and social factors being taken into account (ICRP).

Output phosphor: A layer of material at the exit of an image receptor that emits light when stimulated by electrons.

Patient-entrance dose: The dose delivered to the entrance surface of the patient during a procedure. This will vary from place to place if the beam is moved during the procedure.

Penumbra: The part of a shadow from which some of the light is cut off.

Phantom: A test device simulating radiological properties of a patient.

Photocathode: A layer of material that emits electrons when stimulated by light.

Photoelectric process: A photon transfers its energy to an atomic electron, which is then ejected from the atom with an energy equal to that of the incident photon minus the electron's binding energy. Characteristic X rays are produced as the atomic electrons return to their ground state.

Photoelectrons are also produced when visible light interacts with the electron band structure of certain materials. This latter process is used in photomultiplier tubes and image intensifiers.

Photoelectron: The electron emitted during the photoelectric process.

Photon: A quantum of electromagnetic energy.

Physical format: The physical device (e.g., CD-ROM) used to hold digital information.

Picture archiving and communication system (PACS): A generic term used to describe a (computerized) system for image management.

Pincushion distortion: The geometric distortion of an image that occurs in an image-intensifier when the curved image formed on the input screen is projected onto the flat output screen.

Pixel: The smallest unit in a digital image.

Polychromatic: A beam containing photons of different energy levels (colors).

Primary bean: The X-ray beam entering the patient.

Progressive scanning: A scheme in which the video scan lines are read or written in sequence.

Protective barrier: A structure, such as a wall built to attenuate radiation.

Quality factor: The ratio of the biological effectiveness (per unit dose) of a particular radiation relative to a reference radiation. The quality factors of diagnostic X rays, beta particles, and gamma rays used for brachytherapy are all one.

Quantum sink: The element in an imaging system that involves the fewest information carriers per mm^2. In a well-designed system, the density of information carriers at the quantum sink determines the noise properties of the image.

Radiation: Emission and propagation of electromagnetic energy or decay particles.

Radioactivity: Emission of neutral or charged particles, or electromagnetic radiations from unstable atomic nuclei.

Radiobiology: The study of the biological effects of radiation.

Radiogenic: An effect caused by radiation.

Radiograph: A permanent image produced by passing radiation through an object and detecting the result on a radiosensitive surface.

Radionuclide: An unstable nuclide subject to radioactive decay.

Receptor blur: Image unsharpness caused by the characteristics of the image receptor.

Recoil electron: The electron emerging from a Compton interaction.

Recursive filter: The process of adding a portion of a previous image to a new image.

Redundant array of independent devices (RAID): A set of storage devices with enough redundancy that the failure of any one device does not cause data loss.

Reference dose: A patient entrance dose level for common examinations beyond which justification is required.

Regulation curve: A description of the way in which an X-ray generator controls its output as a function of patient thickness.

Rotating anode: An X-ray tube anode capable of rotating while the tube is in operation.

Scan converter: A device for converting one video format into another.

Scattered radiation: The photons emerging from Compton interactions. These comprise most of the secondary radiation emerging from a patient.

Sensitometric curve: A representation of the response of film to different light or radiation intensities.

Source-to-axis distance (SAD): The distance from the X-ray focal spot to the isocenter of an isocentric imaging system.

Source-to-Image-Receptor distance (SID): The distance from the X-ray focal spot to the entrance surface of the image receptor.

Source-to-skin distance (SSD): The distance from the X-ray focal spot to the skin on the entrance surface the patient.

Spatial filtering: The process of mathematically combining the values of a pixel and its neighbors to affect the visual sharpness of an image.

Spatial resolution: The fineness of detail that can be distinguished in an image.

Stochastic: Involving chance.

Subject contrast: Contrast caused by differential X-ray attenuation of an object and its surroundings.

Suggested state regulations (SSR): A set of model radiation protection regulations periodically published by CRCPD.

System controller: A computer based device controlling the overall function of an X-ray system. Subordinate controllers typically manage specific functions.

Temporal filtering: The process of mathematically combining the values in corresponding pixels in a series of images. This is usually done to minimize the appearance of noise. DSA is a special form of temporal filtering in which subjects common to all of the images in a sequence are subtracted.

Thermionic emission: The emission of electrons from a hot object.

Transformer: A device to transfer electrical energy, usually with a change of voltage.

Transport index (TI): Radiation intensity at one meter from a package of radioactive materials. Used to partially determine the safety of a shipment.

Umbra: The part of a shadow from which all light is cut off.

Unsharp masking: The process of subtracting a blurred version of an image from its original form. The net effect is edge enhancement.

Videodensitometric: The use of the video signal to measure the X-ray absorption properties of an object.

Vidicon: A light-sensitive vacuum tube capable of forming video images.

Vignetting: Radial variation in the intensity of light caused by nonuniform optical performance.

X ray: Electromagnetic radiation produced either by atomic orbital transformations or by the interaction of a charged particle with the electric field of an atom. X-ray photon energies range from a few keV up to several tens of MeV.

X-ray filter: A metal sheet used to change the characteristics of a polychromatic X-ray beam by differential attenuation.

X-ray generator: A set of components arranged to deliver the power and control signals needed to form X-ray images.

Index